DIAGNOSING
—— AND ——
TREATING
MENTAL
ILLNESS

BOOKS IN THE DEMERS BOOKS
HEALTH AND WELL-BEING SERIES

Norma Sawyers-Kurtz, *How to Cope with the Loss of Your Child: A Guide for Grieving Parents* (2010). ISBN: 978-0-9816002-5-3

John V. Wylie, *Diagnosing and Treating Mental Illness: A Guide for Physicians, Nurses, Patients and Their Families* (2010). ISBN: 978-0-9816002-6-0

Eric G. Stephan and R. Wayne Pace, *7 Secrets of a Successful, Tranquil Life: A Guide for People Who Want to Get Out of Hyperdrive* (2010). ISBN 978-0-9816002-7-7

Danny M. O'Dell, *Strength Training for People with Osteoporosis: The Danny O'Dell Method* (2010). ISBN: 978-0-9816002-8-4

OTHER BOOKS OF INTEREST FROM
DEMERS BOOKS AND MARQUETTE BOOKS

John Wheeler, *Last Man Out: Memoirs of the Last Associated Press Reporter Castro Kicked Out of Cuba in the 1960s* (2009). ISBN: 978-0-9816002-0-8

Tom Graves, *Crossroads: The Life and Afterlife of Blues Legend Robert Johnson* (2009). ISBN: 978-0-9816002-1-5

Charles J. Merrill, *Colom of Catalonia: Origins of Christopher Columbus Revealed* (2009). ISBN 978-0-9816002-2-2

John Schulz, Please Don't Do That! The Pocket Guide to Good Writing (2008). ISBN: 978-0-922993-87-1 (booklet)

Phillip J. Tichenor, *Athena's Forum: A Historical Novel* (2005). ISBN: 0-922993-27-0

Melvin DeFleur, *A Return to Innocence: A Novel* (2005). ISBN: 0-922993-50-5

David Demers, *China Girl: One Man's Adoption Story* (2004). ISBN: 0-922993-08-4

DIAGNOSING
—AND—
TREATING
MENTAL
ILLNESS

A Guide for
Physicians,
Nurses,
Patients
and Their
Families

John V. Wylie, M.D.

Demers Books LLC
Spokane, Washington

Printed in the United States of America on acid-free paper.

Library of Congress Cataloging Number
2009906904

ISBN for this Edition
978-0-9816002-6-0

Cover photograph by John Consoli

Books Shown on the Cover

Counsels and Ideals & Selected Aphorisms by William Osler; *The Practice of Behavior Therapy* by Joseph Wolpe; *Cognitive Therapy of Depression* by Aaron Beck, John Rush, Brian Shaw, Gary Emery; *Alcoholics Anonymous Big Book*; *Textbook of Psychopharmacology* by Alan Schatzberg and Charles Nemeroff; *Comprehensive Textbook of Psychiatry*, Volumes 1 & 2 by Benjamin Sadock and Virginia Sadock; *A Treatise on Insanity* by Phillippe Pinel; *The Idea of Phenomenology* by Edmund Husserl; *Basic Writings* by Sigmund Freud; *The Origin of Species & The Descent of Man* by Charles Darwin

Demers Books LLC
3107 East 62nd Avenue
Spokane, Washington 99223
509-443-7057 (voice) / 509-448-2191 (fax)
books@demersbooks.com / www.DemersBooks.com

3 2903 30057 0071

For my patients
and my brother, Bob

CONTENTS

(Continued from the previous page)

PREFACE

Medicine is in my bones. I am a fourth generation physician and started out as a surgeon, my father's esteemed profession. After several years of training, I decided it was not for me. In college, I had majored in the liberal arts and felt the center of my interests were humanistic. After an interim in which I immersed myself in Freud and Jung, I made the decision to train in psychiatry. Although absorbed by the theories of Sigmund Freud, the doctor in my bones was disturbed that they mainly pertained to patients with milder psychiatric conditions. Then, with the arrival of Prozac, it seemed as if the entire edifice of psychoanalysis calved like a glacier into the biochemical soup of the brain.

I have never lost my conviction that, for now and many generations to come, the most accurate descriptions of mental illness derive not from examinations of the brain but from the mouths of patients who suffer from these enigmatic sicknesses. This book consists of what my patients have told me about their illnesses and what made them feel better.

Having pondered the nature of human emotions in health and sickness from many years, I have come to the conclusion that the basic emotions of fear and anger, each exist in pairs and each are in dynamic balance. The fear of being trapped pushes us outward and the fear of separation holds us back. The rage to survive and procreate thrusts us out and the rage granted to the authority of society presses back upon us. Our astonishing abilities to think and speak depend upon the intensity of integration between these interacting emotions; each pair inveighs upon one another both internally and between each other while maintaining equilibrium.

But, just as Icarus[1] flew as close to the sun as possible, it is the sheer volume of these emotional dynamics that, at a certain threshold, also makes them vulnerable to imbalances that cause them to spin out of control. More generally, it is the intensity of emotional reactivities amongst these balanced pairs of emotion that comprise an individual's temperament. A temperament with specific sensitivities can then be pathologically "tuned up" in childhood by certain kinds of stress, or, perhaps, not sufficiently "toughened up" by not enough of certain other kinds of stress. I will never believe that "too much love" causes mental illness. Quite to the contrary, love constructs a sanctuary that, as I have witnessed many times, can sustain a patient through the ravages of these sicknesses whose very existence in our collective mind hides beneath the shroud of our ignorance about them.

Each individual is born with an electronic instrument pre-tuned by the mysteries that braided together its strings to be set in motion by rapidly changing new worlds of experience. Whether who we are as individuals is thrust upon us or chosen by us, mental illness is a part of who we are and how we suffer as a group. Thus, being an intrinsic part of us, we should

---

[1] In Greek mythology, Icarus escaped with his father from an island prison using feathers attached to their shoulders by wax. Icaris wanted to fly higher than he needed to and thereby got too close to the sun, which then melted the wax, and he fell into the sea and drowned.

embrace the mentally ill amongst us and regard them as deserving of our respectful care for paying the price for the soaring genius of our human family.

Chapter 1

THE NATURE OF MENTAL ILLNESS

The term "existential" has been informally adopted by the psychiatric community as an adjective to describe emotional problems experienced by individuals who are basically psychiatrically healthy. The purpose of this Guidebook is to help distinguish existential problems from psychiatric conditions — conditions that should properly be regarded as medical sicknesses — and to provide a concise guide to modern treatments for them. Of course, psychiatry has undergone a major transformation during the past half century with the development of effective medications that are now at the disposal of those primary care physicians who have the inclination to participate in the care of the mentally ill. This book is designed to assist in this participation and as a resource for physicians, nurses, therapists, and patients and their families.

The scientific understanding of the pathophysiology of mental illness lags behind the rest of medicine because of the sheer complexity of the brain. There are no biometric tests for mental illness in clinical use. The fact remains that the most reliable way to diagnose mental illness is to carefully ask the patient to describe how they feel. The Diagnostic and Statistical

Manual of Mental Disorders, or DSM, consists of lists of symptoms for each condition that are heavily dependent on patients' subjective reports of how their experience feels to them. Sigmund Freud and his followers built the entire theory of psychoanalysis on the basis of patients' subjective reports of their emotional experiences. The study of mental function and malfunction by means of examining subjective experience is called *phenomenology* and, although it is a far cry from the concrete certainty of scientific knowledge, in the area of psychiatry it continues to have central relevancy.

Human emotional function is characterized by the interaction of a wide variety of emotions, some of which are in conflict with each another. In health, all these emotions are held in a dynamic balance. It is the thesis of this book that the central theater in which mental illness occurs is at the brain level within which these emotions dynamically and functionally interact. Mental illness occurs when the balance between specific emotions is disrupted. Similar to other complex disorders, the genetic vulnerability to mental illness is diffuse with many genes having small effects, and the biochemistry is a veritable jungle of cause, compensation, and effect. However, trying to understand the genetic basis and microbiology of mental illness before thoroughly understanding the "gross pathology" at the level where emotions functionally interact is like trying to understand the genetics and microbiology of diabetes before understanding the role of insulin.

During the 35 years of my practice as a clinical psychiatrist, I have attempted to assemble a phenomenological theory that specifically distinguishes the aspects of mental conditions which are pathological from those which are existential. In essence, I have tried to give a theoretical structure to the symptoms in the diagnostic manual. Over the years, I have observed how, in each illness, specific normally functioning emotions transform into mental illness, and, when the patient improves, observed how they fit back into their prior normal function. Close attention to how patients describe the subjective effects of psychiatric medications has provided clarification as to the nature of how emotions malfunction in mental illness.

I believe that the pathological transformations undergone by normally functioning emotions are similar to fundamental mechanisms in other medical illnesses that disrupt normal function. For example, mental illness occurs in the brain. The brain is composed of electrochemical circuitry which is regulated by negative feedback controls at many levels. Indeed, the breakdown of feedback regulation from the molecular level all the way up to complex biological processes is surely one of the most fundamental pathological mechanisms in all of medicine.

The simplest examples of negative feedback regulation are hormonal systems in which the substance that stimulates the production of a hormone is inhibited by the hormone itself, such that its level is regulated. In negative feedback, one element stimulates or amplifies another element, which, in turn inhibits or dampens the first. In uncontrolled positive feedback, both elements stimulate or amplify each other. The most commonly experienced example of positive feedback is the squealing of a speaker hooked up to a microphone in a noisy room. The noise is picked up by the microphone, amplified and put out by the speaker; then picked back up by the microphone, around and around up to a squeal (feedback reverberation) until the amplifier is turned down. Most simply put, this is the model I am putting forth as the fundamental phenomenon of mental illness.

Sex is the best gross example of positive feedback. Need I spell out the details? In complex systems, there are positive feedback interactions, which tend to "rev" things up, combined with negative feedback interactions which tend to calm things down. When two people get angry with each other, they act as a positive feedback loop up to the point at which negative feedback controls fail and violence ensues. Similarly, when two people become frightened they too can form a positive feedback loop until negative feedback controls fail and they become hysterical. In mental illness, negative feedback controls on internally interacting emotions fail, releasing them into the squeal of what I will repeatedly refer to as "feedback reverberation." I shall also express this pathology by using the image of emotions "locking up" into feedback reverberation.

The perspective that mental illness represents the release of emotions into uncontrolled hyperactivity is consistent with the science of psychiatry as it is understood so far. Functional imaging of all psychopathology reveals central aspects of neurological hyperactivity across multiple structures of the brain. The fact that vulnerability to mental illness most likely occurs diffusely at the molecular level does not preclude the probability that that the primary locus of the pathology itself exists at high levels of the brain, nor does it preclude secondary effects at the molecular level which not only might contribute to the intransigence of the pathology but also perhaps provide the substrate for intervention with medications and other physical treatments. In short, I firmly believe that a "top down" understanding of mental illness should continue to illuminate a scientific understanding.

The mystery of why these illnesses haven not been swept away long ago by natural selection has lead some to believe that mental illness, at least during some time in the past, served adaptive social functions. As others have suggested, it is possible that some of the genes implicated in mental illness are adaptive in combination with one set of genes but cause mental illness with another set; but I (along with all my patients) am adamant that mental illness, like cancer or any other sickness serves no function for the patient whatsoever and is the enemy of health.

Besides providing a theoretical framework by means of which psychiatric conditions can be differentiated from existential problems, the Guidebook gives a concise compendium of modern treatments for the former. Multiple balances are struck in the presentation of medication treatments, stating general principles whenever possible. Part of the purpose of laying out a comprehensive outline of these treatments is to help the primary care physician make a more informed decision as to the level of complexity at which he or she refers a patient to a psychiatrist or psychotherapist. Effective psychotherapy treatments are described for each condition along with a general sense of how the relationship between the psychotherapist and psychiatrist (or internist) is coordinated.

Finally, I want to convey to any students who might read this book the sense of the excitement I have found in the practice of psychiatry. Since I have been in the field, medication and psychotherapeutic treatments have developed to the point that, with persistence, these painful conditions almost always improve. At the same time, the very nature of these illnesses remains a stubborn mystery. In the daily course of treating patients, the burden of responsibility for this suffering is constantly leavened by the realization that each patient offers another opportunity to view a tantalizing mystery from a slightly different angle. If you are a person with a humanistic bent who also enjoys speculating about mysteries, this is the field for you.

Chapters 1, 3, 4, and 12 give the reader a general understanding of what mental illness is and how it is treated. The section on Panic in chapter 4 is particularly important, because many general principles and medication issues are covered. The other chapters can be read individually as needed.

Chapter 2

WHO SHOULD TREAT MENTAL ILLNESS?

As stated earlier, a principal aim of this book is to sharpen the reader's ability to distinguish the patient with mental illness from people who are suffering from life's inevitable difficulties that lay waiting for us all. I shall return to this crucial distinction repeatedly in many contexts. I feel it is appropriate to use the word "counseling" when referring patients for existential problems, and "treatment" for mental illness. One ought constantly to keep one's "ear to the ground" in search of effective, mental health counselors, particularly those willing to deal with marriages and families. As will be explained, marriages and families, as well as being the source of many existential problems, also can be an inextricable part of mental illness. My experience is that excellent counselors can come from a wide variety of backgrounds including psychology, social work, and the clergy. Many of these counselors have properly clarified the distinction in question by referring to their clients, reserving the word "patient" for those with mental illness.

Traditionally the roles of psychiatrist and therapist were carried out by a single person, but increasingly, these roles are split. It is important to understand that effective psychotherapies have been developed for mental illness and that these treatments have earned practitioners with backgrounds in clinical psychology and social work an indispensable role in treating the mentally ill. Simultaneously, the efficacy of psychiatric medication has also placed psychiatric treatment within reach of the primary care physician. It is the goal of this Guidebook to encourage primary care physicians to participate in the treatment of the mentally ill and one foundation of that participation is to have a firm grasp on the roles of the psychiatrist, the primary physician, and the psychotherapist in modern practice.

In my frequent collaboration with psychotherapists, I have found it not of utmost importance to declare who is in charge with ultimate authority, which is of interest principally to lawyers in assessing blame. In modern practice, it is more and more common for a psychotherapist see the patient most frequently, say once a week, and a psychiatrist to be in a specialist, consultant role, seeing the patient only as frequently as demanded by the activity of the symptoms. Because of the length and flux of these professional relationships, the need for communication varies frequently and is usually carried on by phone rather than by formal letters.

Primary care physicians are by far in the best position to make referrals to specialists simply because they can see and hear the results of treatment when the patients come back for their regular checkups. Not only should the physician have a ready list of psychiatrists and therapists who have various subspecialty training and interests, but to refine the list as to kinds of patient personalities various mental health care providers are particularly adept at treating. On the other hand, both psychiatrists and psychotherapists have also sifted through their counterparts with whom they work effectively and also can make a subsequent, secondary referral. Indeed, conversations between primary care physicians and trusted mental health care providers as to whom would be effective for a given patient are always appropriate.

If you are an internist who enjoys helping psychiatric patients as I do, I feel you should go ahead and conduct the medical end of psychiatric treatment, preferably with a therapist also seeing the patient. I certainly have enjoyed the collegial role of "curbside" consultant to many of my physician friends and was always happy to either formally consult or take over the treatment for a while if things were not working out. To those physicians particularly interested in treating psychiatric patients, I strongly recommend the excellent comprehensive text on the subject, *Psychiatry for Primary Physicians* published by the American Medical Association Press.

The psychiatrist has specific expertise and retains authority in the area of diagnosing mental illness. However, the stigma still attached to mental illness also adheres to the psychiatrist. It will not infrequently be encountered in the form of resistance to a recommended referral. The response to this resistance should be firm. The experience of seeing a psychiatrist should be no different from that of consulting any other medical specialist. The qualities are the same: kindliness, the ability to listen, the flexibility to entertain more than one diagnosis, and to know when to seek further consultation, especially if treatments are not working.

Furthermore, the psychiatrist, now more securely back in the role of physician, has reclaimed the power to confer the status of patienthood with all its ancient rights and privileges. I generally like to have the patient bring the spouse or a family member to the first visit mainly to corroborate the history after meeting alone with the patient. After a diagnosis of mental illness has been made, when possible and appropriate, I have made it a practice to talk to the family about granting the same, full privileges of being deemed a patient as would be given those suffering from physical sicknesses. There is a respectful care associated with the designation of being a patient that addresses the isolation inherent in all illness. My patients have often spoken to me about the loneliness of mental illness. As my physician father used to say: "There should be no shame in sickness."

Chapter 3

PATHOLOGICAL ANXIETY

Anxiety is the most common psychiatric condition. Once in a while I will run into someone who doesn't understand the concept of anxiety. Anxiety is fear that something bad has or is going to happen. For most people, anxiety is a robustly healthy emotion which motivates us to live cautious, prudent, hardworking lives. As I have told my patients over the years, "Most people get up and go to work each day not because they want to, but because they are afraid of the consequences if they don't." Because anxiety is such an emotional staple of normal life, defining a boundary beyond which it becomes a disorder is all the more challenging.

The phenomenon of Panic shall be presented first because it is the prototypical example of the primary pathological process shared by all mental illness as presented in the introduction: the failure of negative feedback controls resulting in runaway feedback reverberation. In Panic, specific anxieties increase in intensity up to a threshold beyond which they degenerate into feedback reverberation in which the constituent emotions are locked into a high-pitched emotional runaway circuitry. Panic lurks as the potential pathological culmination of all other anxiety conditions and, thus, provides unifying context for a general discussion of the nature and treatments of anxiety, particularly a detailed description of medication therapies.

Following the lengthy discussion of Panic, two other anxiety conditions, Phobias and Generalized Anxiety Disorder, will be briefly discussed along with the treatment considerations unique to them. This section is followed by a very personal philosophical discussion about existential anxiety. The Chapter ends with a discussion of hysteria including advice about what to do if someone is threatening to commit suicide. Obsessive Compulsive Disorder and Post-Traumatic Stress Disorder are also anxiety disorders, but shall be presented later in the book, because their distinctive natures places them outside of the broad theme of Chapters 3 and 4 of demonstrating the relationship between anxiety and depression.

PANIC: THE NEXUS OF ANXIETY

Think of being in an airplane that suddenly loses altitude. A rush of adrenalin surges up from your stomach into your chest and throat as you clutch your chair and attempt to hold onto, really, yourself. Now imagine that same experience happening "out of the blue" — such as when you are sleeping or walking down the street. The first thought is that some internal catastrophe has occurred, such as a heart attack or stroke. Even after having suffered many panic episodes, it is difficult not to believe while it is happening that something catastrophic and fatal has happened or is about to.

The escalation of anxiety into panic serves as a general, overall example of how normal emotional function transforms into emotional illness. Every one of us will panic if the circumstances are extreme enough, but whatever function panic may serve in those rare cases would be happily forfeited by the legions of patients who are relentlessly seized by this emotional inferno for no apparent reason. Often the initial episode of panic is in reaction to a confluence of stresses in a young person's life, but that initial experience is so shatteringly traumatic that the passage of time becomes saturated with the dread of its impending repetition. In a cruel and vicious cycle the anxious anticipation of the recurrence of panic brings it on all the more intensely.

WHAT PANIC TELLS US ABOUT ANXIETY

Because of its pure intensity, the experience of panic must be examined closely in order to clarify the nature of its ingredients of anxiety, which are normally concealed by their blending into the flowing mixture of normal emotional life. In mental illness, the constituents of interacting emotions, "pop themselves out" and, despite their shrill distortion, reveal the basic aspects of their composition. A basic duality in the human mind clearly emerges in firsthand descriptions of the exquisite suffering of panic: "I become anxious, and then I become anxious about being anxious." One half of the person makes the other half anxious in an escalating spiral. Within panic the two fundamental human anxieties are pitted against one another.

TWO ANXIETIES: BEING TRAPPED AND ABANDONED

The most basic human fear is that of being trapped or even suffocated. I often refer patients to the image of a "rat in a trap" preoccupied by escape. Surely, one reason that the nation was so gripped by the 9/11 attacks on the World Trade Center was that everyone could instinctively relate to the specific horror of being trapped. People who are prone to panic do not like hot, humid weather. "It feels like a hot blanket covering me up." The fear of being trapped goes well beyond a physical circumstance but is a fundamental emotional component to one's social circumstances. Humans can feel trapped by their jobs, their economic or social status, and let's not leave out families and marriages. Poor humans! We have to constantly balance our fear of being trapped with our other major fear.

The next most basic fear in humans is separation anxiety. Once an attachment has been established, particularly a family or romantic bond, the emotional rupture of that connection produces anxiety. Who among you cannot recall from your childhood a circumstance or two when you were seized with anxiety in response to the departure of a parent or some other person with whom you had established a close attachment? People who are prone to anxiety problems in general are especially sensitive to separation such that, often mere physical separation, for example a child or a spouse going on a trip produces excessive anxiety. Separation anxiety can also be manifested in response to physical circumstances, such as traveling even if everyone is going with you. If you are afraid of spiders, it is much worse to see one in your room alone than outside when you are with a friend.

Whereas, in normal functioning, these two anxieties balance and weave together the avoidance of life's many traps with the maintenance of family bonds and friendships, in the illness of panic they suddenly coil together and rise up like a serpent.

PHYSICAL SYMPTOMS IN PANIC

One discovers the true nature of panic only after following many patients with this disorder over long periods of time. Initially, the experience of panic triggers physical symptoms, such as rapid heart rate and the feeling of suffocation causing compensatory over breathing, which, in turn, can cause numbness and tingling. Often, the patient focuses on these symptoms thinking some dire physical illness, such as a heart attack or a stroke, has stricken her and she is about to die. The normal trusting relationship with one's body, including gut reliance that changes in the basic rhythm of heart rate and breathing reflect either physical exertion or some real danger in one's environment is fundamentally disrupted. Patients are reassured by initial visits to a physician or emergency room, which prompt resolution of the panic symptoms with a dose of a benzodiazepine tranquilizer. As treatment progresses, and the physical symptoms abate, patients often first realize that the root panic experience is separate from those physical symptoms that had initially appeared to cause it but had actually just exacerbated it.

SHOULD PATIENTS CHANGE THEIR LIVES OR TREAT THE ILLNESS

The basic answer to this question is to treat the illness. Panic Disorder can be precipitated by a single event, in which case the section on Post-Traumatic Stress Disorder (PTSD) should be read in Chapter 7. Most often the initial episode of panic is in the context of an ongoing circumstance, such as a job or a relationship, in which the patient feels more and more trapped but afraid to leave. Think about how broad a swath that situation is in life, particularly in the younger years.

In panic, the fear of being trapped triggers the fear of separation in the vicious feedback reverberation cycle characteristic of all mental illness. Perhaps the initial episode is an indication that the current circumstance is, indeed, beyond the tolerance of the patient's sensitivities, and, therefore consideration should be given as to extraction from it. Great care must be exercised in making such a decision however, because, very rapidly, the patient's view becomes distorted such that the confining nature of any commitment creates anxiety and the possibility of further episodes of panic.

The stock and trade of those in mental health care, ever growing with experience, is a sense of the kinds of basic life experience that are fundamentally and "existentially" upsetting. A careful calculation should be made in which the shadow cast by the reality of the circumstance is weighed against the patient's heightened sensitivities to it. Whether or not the decision is made to leave the ongoing circumstance, the panic symptoms must be treated directly as an illness.

CAUSES OF PANIC: GENES VS. CHILDHOOD UPBRINGING

Yes, I recommend giving medication "up front" for panic. Inevitably, this advice begs the question as to whether this means that the condition is a "chemical imbalance." I respond by informing patients that all the unique emotional reactions that combine to comprise their particular temperament ultimately have physical and chemical roots. I point out to them that in a spectrum of emotional dispositions in the population, they are on the more anxious and sensitive side. Most of these patients have figured that out by themselves already, and I confirm that these qualities are not pathological in and of themselves.

Asked whether the condition is "all genetic," I respond that all mental illness is roughly 50 percent genetic and 50 percent environment. I ruefully add that we have not made much progress in understanding the actual nature of the interaction between genes and childhood experiences, except that it is much more complicated than we used to think. I ask whether any of the patient's relatives are "high strung," reassuring them that they "come by this honestly" when they tell me that, indeed, some are.

There are two simple examples of how genes and childhood experience could theoretically interact. A genetically anxious parent could respond to their genetically anxious child by either over protection or pushing too hard, in either case possibly making the anxiety problem worse. I find that knowledge of this sort never helps to control the active symptoms of panic and sometimes compromises the needed support of key family members by the implication that they are responsible for the problem. Quite to the contrary, I try not to fail to reassure the patient and the family that panic is not a result of faulty child rearing or even abuse, which leaves a far more complex footprint primarily manifested by disruptions in abilities to carry on close relationships. If the patient and the family are interested in speculating about the interaction between "constitutional" anxiety and the childhood culture of the patient, that is best done later by a therapist perhaps with an eye towards altering responses to excessive anxiety in the patient's own children.

TREATMENT OF PANIC AND PATHOLOGICAL ANXIETY

With wry humor, I have repeatedly told my patients with Panic that the best treatment for anxiety is to not be anxious. What I mean by this is that getting on top of a panic disorder is a "confidence game." When panic strikes several times, the patient is placed in the anxious position of anticipating "when the other shoe will drop" which, in the cruel signature of mental illness, brings on the condition even more. So, if by "hook or crook" (drugs) the panic can be controlled for a period of weeks or months, the patient's anticipation that it will reoccur at any given moment will naturally decrease, bringing with it a return of confidence which then collapses this particular vicious cycle and replaces it with a healthy one. Treatment in psychiatry is often slow, and one of its most active ingredients is persistence. Patients under psychiatric treatment must become scientists and continually measure their own symptom episodes in 3 basic ways: *frequency, intensity,* and *duration.* How often does it occur, how bad was it, and how long did it last. Is it getting better, worse, or staying the same.

1. *Insight Oriented Psychotherapy*

Until 30 years ago, all psychiatric patients were treated with Insight Oriented Psychotherapy. These treatments use Freudian concepts to help patients develop insight into the manner in which repressed childhood feelings continue to influence their adult emotional life in adverse ways.

Many patients have told me that they have benefited from the self-knowledge resulting from this procedure which had added depth and meaning to their emotional lives. In order for this psychotherapy to be effective, it needs to be administered in hour long sessions at least once a week, over several years. Because of this intensive use of medical resource for a single patient, this type of therapy has progressively been squeezed economically. For the illnesses described in this Guidebook, I feel that Insight Oriented Psychotherapy continues to be the primary treatment modality in the two conditions in which lack of insight is a major feature: persistent hysteria (described at the end of this chapter) and Borderline Personality Disorder (described in Chapter 5). It shall be mentioned below that Generalized Anxiety Disorder is another condition for which this treatment should be considered. Otherwise, Insight Oriented Psychotherapy seems to be most effective for emotional problems, which are below the threshold of illness as defined in this book, but it can be helpful in consolidating gains in some after these illnesses have been treated. I have never discouraged my patients from pursuing this form of treatment, but have warned them that I have seen long term, intensive psychotherapy become a "hiding place" in which commitments in one's real life are compromised. I generally feel that relationship problems should be treated conjointly in psychotherapy with the spouse and/or family involved.

In response to the need for more "targeted," results-oriented treatments for specific conditions emphasized in this guidebook that do meet the criteria for illness, several other modalities have proven to be effective.

2. *Cognitive Therapy*

Cognitive therapy is a relatively new psychological treatment in which patients' attitudes or "belief systems" about themselves are the focus of treatment. In cognitive therapy, entrenched faulty beliefs, such as "everyone thinks I am a loser" are challenged as to their accuracy. These kinds of faulty belief systems can increase anxiety to thresholds which release panic and therapeutically altering them can help prevent its recurrence.

Cognitive therapy has become an important adjunctive tool with proven effectiveness, particularly in the treatment of the full spectrum of depression including those deemed illnesses as shall be discussed. But it is of vital importance that the patient maintains the correct belief that the panic phenomenon, itself, is a true illness that has torn itself away from pre-existing belief systems whether or not they were faulty. Panic is attributable to the breakdown of emotional regulation at a more fundamental psychological level than belief. Once mental illness has been diagnosed, it is a grave error to imply to patients that they are "doing it to themselves," because this false belief can lead to stigmatic attitudes toward mental illness typified by the exhortation to "snap out of it."

3. *Behavioral (Desensitization) Therapy*

The other main adjunctive psychological treatment is desensitization, which falls under the rubric of Behavioral Therapy. The therapeutic effect of desensitization on anxiety has been proven so many times that it approaches the status of a therapeutic Law. That Law states that, over the long run, if the patient is anxious in response to some identifiable object or situation, such as being in a grocery store, avoiding the store makes the anxiety worse, while exposing oneself to it in measured steps makes it worse at first, but, with persistent exposure, makes it better.

If you are afraid of bridges, first think about bridges, then go watch them from a distance, then slowly creep out onto one and sit out there, not for a couple of minutes, but for a couple of hours. But again, it is important to realize that, like cognitive therapy, desensitization is a treatment for anxiety, not panic. In carefully managing the pace of exposure to the anxiety-provoking circumstance, it is important to remain well below the panic level, which, if exceeded, sets back the treatment. As shall be discussed, Behavioral Therapy is the primary treatment modality for all phobias and Obsessive Compulsive Disorder. Although the root panic phenomenon is not treatable through desensitization, the anxieties which precipitate it in the first place, as well as those secondarily caused by it, can be.

For example, in Panic, the "insult to injury" increased anxiety caused by the above-mentioned physical symptoms of "air hunger" and rapid pulse can be helped by desensitizing the patient to them. In a calm, secure situation the patient is instructed to over-breathe in order to reproduce the symptoms of numbness and tingling, or to exercise to increase the pulse, then stop and try to relax in the face of these experiences.

Commonly patients with Panic Disorder have panic level responses to being "trapped" in specific closed-in spaces (claustrophobia) such as elevators, subways, airplanes, crowded theaters, etc. Alternatively or additionally, panic can be released by being out and separated from home. Once the panic phenomenon is under control with medications, the therapeutic agenda of nudging the patient into attempting to gradually increase exposure to these environments must immediately commence. Because the fundamental dynamic in all pathological anxiety disorders is becoming "anxious about being anxious," I have often given these patients the curious advice to, "Pick a tolerable level of anxiety, and try to desensitize yourself to becoming anxious in response to that baseline level." I don't really think that this actually works, but the advice serves to illustrate dual the nature of their condition.

4. *Self-Relaxation, Biofeedback, Meditation, and Yoga*

I have tried to emphasize to all of my patients with anxiety disorders the importance of establishing a routine whereby, several times per day, they take at least 10 minutes during which they attempt to relax. The secret of relaxing is that it takes mental effort and concentration. Concentrate on your breathing: slow it down and control it. Then concentrate on relaxing the jaw, neck and shoulder muscles (visualize a coat hanger with the hook being your jaw muscles, twisted perpendicular to the hanger, which is the back of your neck and your shoulder muscles).

Like any physical discipline program, it helps to have a trainer. Relaxation therapists, who, sadly, are a dying breed, use biofeedback machines. Electrodes are adhered to the patient's forehead with wires attached to a machine which transduces the level of muscle tension to a display on a TV monitor. Patients obtain immediate feedback on whether their efforts at relaxing are successful and thus can more quickly learn how to do it. I certainly encourage any of the Eastern forms of meditation and particularly the daily practice of yoga for patients with anxiety conditions. It is important to understand that the benefits from these regular activities are not immediate and results should not be expected for at least 6 weeks. The benefits from these modalities may not be decisive without other psychiatric treatment, but they are absolutely reliable if the patient persists in practicing them over the course of months and years.

5. Medications[2] in the Treatment of Panic and Pathological Anxiety

Again, the best treatment for panic is to block the panic decisively for a period of not days, not years, but months. Two classes of drugs are approved for the treatment of panic: benzodiazepine tranquilizers and the Serotonin Reuptake Inhibitors (SSRI's) antidepressants. Please allow me to digress into a mini-tirade: Valium (available as diazepam), Prozac (available as fluoxetine), Thorazine (available as chlorpromazine) and lithium were all prototypes of their particular class, and all have "hit the media" in their day resulting in all being tarnished by the stigma of mental illness. You would casually comment that you are on an antibiotic, but to tell someone you are taking one of these "bad boys" is an entirely different matter. Nevertheless, these have been extraordinarily important medicines. Before Valium, the barbiturate sleeping pills, such as Seconal, were the only tranquillizing medications available, which could and frequently did cause death in even mild overdose, especially with alcohol.

---

[2]If I use a brand name for the purpose of recognizability, I will always put the generic name in parenthesis and note if it is available at the time of publication.

Benzodiazepines (Valium derivatives) can be fatal in huge overdose in conjunction with alcohol, but rarely benzodiazepines alone. Although both barbiturates and benzodiazepines are addictive, a sudden cessation of barbiturates is much more lethal. Stopping barbiturates can precipitate Status Epilepticus (a constant epileptic seizure). Seizures are also a threat when benzodiazepines are suddenly stopped, but much less of a threat.

All treatment interventions have up and down sides. The up side of benzodiazepine tranquilizers is that they work both reliably and quickly (within 15-45 minutes) to suppress not only the panic, but also the "anticipatory" anxiety that one is about to have a panic attack. Reliability is the main benefit. Once panic disordered patients take a tranquilizer, they know that the "cavalry will soon appear over the hill." It is a general rule with all psychiatric drugs, except in dire emergencies, that patients should be begin a course of drugs with small doses, usually one half of the minimum available dose, obtained by simply cutting the pill in half. Understandably, anxiety patients tend to be anxious about any alteration of their mental status, which is already unbearably altered. The first dose is taken in the evening, early enough for the patient to get a sense of what the response is before going to sleep. The art of taking tranquilizers consists of slowly increasing the dose up to strike an appropriate balance between the continuance of anxiety if the dose is too small and sedation if it is too high.

If the frequency of panic level anxiety is low enough, or in patients who have discontinued all medication after successful treatment, an acceptable option is to take tranquilizers only occasionally. The patient might only take an appropriate dose in anticipation of entering into a situation, such as flying, that has triggered panic or anxiety in the past. Furthermore, once it crosses the person's "radar screen" that anxiety is being triggered and starting to escalate into panic, the earlier the patient takes the medicine, the better: "Cut it off at the pass!" Often, just the comfort of knowing that the pill is tucked in the patient's wallet or purse and "it's there if I need it" is sufficient. The mantra I give my patients when thinking about psychiatric medicines in general in order to inoculate them against stigmatic attitudes is that they are a "tool, not a crutch." Nevertheless, addiction is a very real problem with tranquilizers.

Let there be no doubt that benzodiazepine tranquillizers can be addicting, and this should be understood by all who take them. Some of the tranquilizers are inherently more addictive than others, but all have addictive potential if taken more frequently than several times a week for longer than a month or so. Physical withdrawal after long-standing dependence on tranquilizers can be, in the words of several of my patients who have gone through it, "a bitch." Not only does the anxiety come back, but it is accompanied by muscular spasm and insomnia.

The secret of getting off benzodiazepine tranquillizers is to do it very, very slowly and methodically. My patients get very good at cutting up pills into halves and quarters. I tell them, "Get out your jeweler's lens." If a patient is on a high dose, often they can make larger reductions at the beginning of the program, but then need to slow down later. I point out that reducing a 5 mg dose to 4 mg is only a 20 percent reduction, whereas reducing a 2 mg dose by the same 1 mg is a 50 percent reduction. Sometimes, to emphasize the point that the slower the reduction the better, I tell patients that it can take half the time that they have been on a tranquillizer to get off of it. Usually patients want to go faster and I relent to their impatience, but the point has been made and received.

Now, after having said all that, I also emphasize that, in addition to physical dependency and consequent withdrawal, there is one other component to addiction. This is the idea of drug abuse. Benzodiazepines can be abused because some people enjoy their effects as a "high." In general, patients with anxiety disorders do not abuse drugs, because they are "high enough" with their anxiety. As I have often put it, anxiety patients are not trying to "get off" (high), they are trying to get "back on" (feel back to normal). Just as physical addiction to narcotics is not as severe when patients are taking them properly for unbearable pain, tranquilizers taken for unbearable anxiety or panic do not produce the same level of addiction as they might to an abuser.

Xanax (available as: alprazolam) is by far the most addicting of the benzodiazepine group. This is due both to the fact that it is inherently more potent than most of the others, but more because it has a shorter half life, which is the time a drug takes to reduce to half of its peak blood level. More relevant to patients, is the clinical half life of a drug, which is simply the time elapsed as reported by the patient between when it starts and then stops having an effect. The clinical half life of alprazolam is about 4 to 5 hours, after which the resurgence of anxiety reminds the patient that he or she needs to take another pill in order to feel calm. It is not a good mentality to establish a pattern of having to take a pill because you can feel the effects of the last one wearing off. That has the "earmarks" of addiction. A long-acting formulation of Xanax partially solves this "roller coaster" problem by slowly releasing the medication over a longer period of time, but you are still stuck with the same short half life drug which drops off just as quickly if you miss a twice daily dose. On the other hand, alprazolam is probably the most powerful anti-anxiety, anti-panic drug, so it could be used in the short term for very severe, intractable cases. Otherwise, I feel it is well to keep alprazolam doses in an addiction-comfort-zone neighborhood of ¼ mg several times a day. Nevertheless, in some cases, a short half life drug may be helpful.

Ativan (available as lorazepam), in my opinion, is the mildest of the benzodiazepine tranquilizers. Although its half-life is about as short as alprazolam, it is not nearly as powerful a drug, and therefore not as addicting. A short half-life drug can be a distinct advantage, particularly in the elderly, because the level of the drug does not build up in the system over time. Because it is metabolized outside of the liver, it is "cleaner" in that there are fewer interactions with other medications, with the obvious exception of alcohol. ("If you've taken a tranquillizer, you've already had a drink!") Nevertheless, in doses of 2 mg or higher, larazepam's short half life means that the patient must be vigilant about situations in which he or she might suddenly stop taking it, such as forgetting to take it on a trip, or during an unexpected hospitalization. But, all and all, lorazepam is one of my preferred choices of tranquillizers, particularly for the elderly.

Clonazepam is my favorite choice for pathological anxiety conditions in general. But first, the bad news. Some years ago, I consulted on two elderly patients in the hospital who were virtually unresponsive and both looked as if they had had a stroke. However, their common problem turned out to be long-standing doses of clonazepam which had simply "caught up with them" and conked them out. Both of these patients woke up and were fine after reducing the dose. But other than this dose-build-up problem, I generally prefer clonazepam in the treatment of anxiety. It is well tolerated by patients because it is potent and has a half-life that is long enough to enable patients to take it only 2 times a day without the up and down "roller coaster" effect of having to urgently take the next dose because the last one is wearing off. The clinical half-life is about 8-10 hours so that the ups and downs of both the onset and withdrawal of a given dose are hardly perceptible and thus minimizes the addictive potential. As I shall repeat in the section on addiction, a substance is addictive in direct relation to its speed of onset. That is why the "quick hit" of nicotine in cigarette smoking is so addictive. Still, after taking even 1 mg of clonazepam per day for long periods of time, the patient needs to be withdrawn slowly. Incidentally, it is standard practice to shift over to clonazepam from an equivalent dose of a shorter half-life tranquillizer and then initiate withdrawal due to greater ease and margin of safety. Like all psychiatric medication, I start with a small dose and then build it up to hit the happy medium between anxiety and sedation, as mentioned above.

For some reason, in medicine, the first drug that is discovered in a general class usually "hangs in there" through all the subsequent minor alterations of the chemical compound that produce "improved" copy-cat drugs and maintains some role in treatment. *Valium* (available as diazepam) is no exception. Unique amongst all benzodiazepines, *diazepam* has a direct muscle relaxant property, so it is used for muscle spasms, such as those of the back. But this same property is a negative characteristic for chronic administration, because, after taking it for a while, it makes one feel like a "wet noodle-jelly fish" and tends to depress patients. It also is more easily abused because, although it has a long half-life, it is absorbed very rapidly into the brain, and, therefore, is quickly perceptible in as short as 10-15 minutes after ingestion as a sudden feeling of relaxation.

However, this initial "spike" effect also makes it an ideal "fire extinguisher" to quickly extinguish a panic attack in its early take-off stage. My advice in prescribing it is something like the following: "If you are out in the middle of nowhere, just put it in your mouth and chew it up and then know you will be fine in 15 minutes (but not while driving)." Before using this medication, I have patients "test drive" several doses in non-stressful situations, when they are going to be at home for the rest of the day so they can familiarize themselves to how a given dose effects them. I do not want patients to have any uncertainty about what a drug is going to do in a "commando" panic circumstance. I have many patients walking around with a few vintage, crumbling diazepam tablets in their wallets. If I see them, I remind them that, unlike wine, medications usually don't get better with age so I write them a fresh prescription for 5 tablets to last them another couple of years.

Prozac (available as fluoxetine), which was introduced in 1988, is by far the most important medication in psychiatry since I began training in 1972. Patients who, sometimes for decades, had been dutifully pouring out their hearts on psychoanalysts' couches (which continue to be the object of stigmatic ridicule in cartoons) suddenly felt "normal" after starting Prozac. Shortly thereafter, Paxil (available as paroxetine) and Zoloft (available as sertlaline) followed, and then Celexa (available as citalopram), Lexapro (generic: escitalopram), and Effexor XR (avalablie as venlafaxin XR[3]). Not so well known is that, several years after Prozac was approved by the FDA for the treatment of depression, it was demonstrated that these drugs were just as effective for anxiety and panic. Wellbutrin SR (available as bupropion SR[4]), an antidepressant with very different biochemical effects, was also approved by the FDA for depression about the same time as Prozac but does not have these benefits in anxiety/panic conditions.

As implied in the name, the central effect of the SSRI's is to increase the amount of serotonin in synapses widely distributed in the brain. I have come to feel, again through talking to my patients over the years, that the effect of raising the level of brain serotonin is primarily to reduce anxiety, which then, as I will discuss later, secondarily improves depression. My patients have repeatedly told me that the SSRI drugs simply decrease the intensity of their emotional reactions to stressful situations at the time they

---

[3] The long acting form, venlafaxin XR (extended release), is preferred
[4] The long acting form, bupropion SR (sustained release), is preferred.

are occurring. "I had been stressed out by my boss who's a yeller, and losing my temper with my kids. He is still yelling, and they are still misbehaving, but it is all simply not getting to me as much."

Patients with pathological anxiety are high strung, sensitive, and generally "emotional" (a characteristic which I generally like.) I tell my patients that emotional sensitivity is the "ticket of admission" to get into my office. No insensitive people are allowed in here. In the population out there, there is a bell curve with respect to how emotionally reactive people are to the events of their lives. Some people, found on the left side of the curve, do not react that much. Most people who experience panic can be found on the hyper-reacting right side of the curve. It seems to me that the basic constitutional vulnerability to mental illness in general is high emotional reactivity. The best single adjective that I have come up with to describe the effect of the Prozac-type serotonin drugs is "buffer": they should be referred to as "emotional buffers" rather than antidepressants.

There are two reasons why it is difficult to ascertain whether antidepressants are working. First of all, it takes a while before the therapeutic effect "kicks in": up to 2 or even 3 weeks. I call this the "Alan Greenspan factor." As Chairman of the Federal Reserve Board, he used to raise the interest rates, and no one knew what impact it was going to have on the economy for many months. In the case of antidepressants, it is weeks not months. Occasionally, it works in several days and, rarely, immediately, like the tranquillizers. I tell my patients that, like the rest of life, the bad stuff (side-effects) happen "up front" and you have to wait for the good stuff. Most common are temporary side effects such as a little bit of jitteriness or gastrointestinal "queasiness" which go away in several days. Like all psychiatric medicines (I am a stickler about this), they should be started at ½ the lowest dose available (if it is a capsule, have the patient open it up and dump ½ of it out and put it back together) for several days until the patient is confident that any side-effects are tolerable.

The second reason it is difficult to tell whether SSRI medications are working is that, when they do work, nothing "positive" is happening. They do not make you feel good; they make you feel less bad. Patients often are surprised to discover, almost as an "after-thought," that, when in a situation that is normally very stressful, they find that the level of stress is significantly reduced. Droves of my patients have described the effect as feeling "back to normal," or even, "I feel normal for the first time," or "Now I know what normal is." That these drugs are mind-restoring, rather than mind-altering is the reason these medications have no addiction potential, one of their principal virtues.

Antidepressants, like all treatments in medicine, have their down sides. First of all, patients are compelled to take a pill every single day, not just when the anxiety crops up. So if a patient has a panic/anxiety problem that occurs only once a month or less, he or she is better off taking tranquillizers only when the problem occurs, or even better, in advance of a situation that the patient anticipates will bring on an anxiety attack. Although antidepressants are not addictive and no one is selling them on the streets to get high, if one remains on them in some cases longer than 3-4 months or, for almost everyone, for over a year (which is often recommended), a person must take at least a month, preferably several, to wean off of them. It is not medically dangerous to stop them abruptly, but so-called "discontinuation" effects can be extremely uncomfortable for some patients. As in the case when beginning the medication, physical side-effects of withdrawal precede any relapse of psychiatric symptoms. These withdrawal reactions are most often dizziness, sometimes described as "head rushes," or more generalized flu-like symptoms which may necessitate extremely gradual tapering off of the medication over several months. Similar to the tranquillizers, short half-life antidepressants, such as *Paxil* (available as paroxetine) and *Effexor XR* (available as venlafaxin XR), can be more difficult to get off than the others and this is one reason not to use either as first choices.

The most complained-about side effect of antidepressants is that they do the same thing to patients' sex lives as they do to their emotional life. They make most people less reactive sexually, most commonly making it more difficult reach an orgasm, but also decreasing the sex drive itself (libido). Lack of sexual motivation can be tough on some relationships but also, occasionally, good for others. Another "class effect" of the SSRI antidepressant drugs is that they can cause weight gain, particularly in patients who struggle with their weight prior to taking the medication. Weight gain can be counteracted by diet and exercise, but it commonly adds one more degree of difficulty.

Very occasionally, some patients have complained that the primary effect of the SSRI antidepressants dampens their emotional life experience somewhat. However, with the benefit of gradual fluctuation of the dose up and down to "test the waters," most usually decide that the trade-off is worth it. An amusing anecdote places the SSRI effect "on the money": A friend (not a patient) of mine, who is a fanatic Knick fan from New York, woke me up with his cell-phone one night from Madison Square Garden ranting that his doctor had put him on Prozac and it had turned him into an "out-of-towner." No hysterics at the slam-dunks.

The administration of psychiatric drugs is an inexact science and there are many valid treatment protocols. Much of the following is subjective clinical impression, familiar in the "shop talk" among psychiatrists, but, perhaps, not so to other physicians. Prozac (available as fluoxetine) is the granddaddy of SSRI's. Because it has been around the longest, it is the most tested and we have the most experience with it. This translates into a higher comfort level in unusual situations, such as in the use of extremely high doses (over 100mg) in someone whose anxiety is uncontrolled by more normal doses. It is also preferred in pregnancy due to a larger data base than the others. Taking SSRI's during pregnancy remains controversial in the field and pregnancy-aged women need to know that they are not completely free of complications. In fact, a conversation about effects in pregnancy should be part of the discussion before prescribing any drug to women in that age group. I have occasionally seen significant weight gain with fluoxetine and the rare "pooping out" of its therapeutic effect is a recognized phenomenon. I rarely use Paxil (available as paroxetine) early in treatment because of the short-half life discontinuation problem, because it appears to cause more weight gain and sometimes daytime fatigue. On the other hand, paroxetine is the least likely to cause gastrointestinal distress (most SSRI's can occasionally cause diarrhea) and, at high doses (40-50mg), it has the most proven efficacy for anxiety when other SSRI trials do not work. As mentioned earlier, due to anticipated discontinuation problems, I use *Effexor XR* (available as venlafaxin XR) only after I have tried other anti-depressants. As a first choice SSRI, I usually give either *Zoloft* (available as sertraline), which is slightly energizing, citalopram (which is a generic), or *Lexapro* (generic: ecitalopram), which is a "purified" (the active isomer) form of citalopram and not yet available as a generic. I use *Cymbalta* (generic duloxetine), a newer antidepressant, as a "second line" choice particularly if sedation is part of the clinical picture. *Cymbalta* is chemically similar to *Effexor XR* but seems easier to establish a correct dose and has fewer discontinuation problems.

Many patients have been taking Prozac or its equivalents since 1988, and there have been no serious long-term effects, such as cancer or dementia, and if any-one does determine that there is even a hint of a problem, you can bet that it will be big news. I have occasionally pointed out to patients who are suspicious of psychiatric medication and concerned about their long term effects, that having 5 or 10 years (or a lifetime) of untreated panic/anxiety disorder is definitely not healthy, not to mention diminishment in quality of life. Hints of this are implied in highly publicized studies demonstrating chronic anxiety causing shrinkage of the hippocampus in the brain.

Finally, I should not fail to mention the issue of SSRI's perhaps causing "suicidal thinking" in children. I am not a child psychiatrist, and thus have next to no experience with children. Children react to psychiatric medication somewhat differently than do adults. It seems to me children are more prone to hysteria (see discussion below), and that psychotherapy with family involvement is almost always indicated when children are being treated. Nevertheless psychiatric medications are frequently indicated and I generally feel there is more prejudice in withholding them than giving them. In the little experience I have had, I have always insisted that a parent be intimately involved in the administration and monitoring of medications in children even up through the teenage years. With apologies to this group, teenagers are generally not that great when it comes to remembering to take pills.

The rule in psychiatry, as in the rest of medicine, is to start with the least invasive (harmful side-effects) treatment and to allow the persistent strength of the illness to call forth the strength and further invasiveness of additional treatments. I would place on a continuum from least invasive to most: the intermittent use of tranquillizers, then taking one of the SSRI drugs, if necessary up to a high level; then daily use of a tranquillizer (which can be done simultaneously with an SSRI), and then, if these are not getting it done, the brief or intermittent use of a major tranquillizer.

Major tranquillizers are drugs approved for the treatment of Schizophrenia, which primarily alter the dopamine neurotransmitter systems in the brain. Two original drugs in this class of medicines were *Thorazine* and *Haldol,* which, although revolutionary when they were first discovered, caused symptoms of Parkinson's Disease, hard to treat tremors, and sometimes, with over use, were criticized for turning patients into "zombies." Developed in the past 15 years, a new class of these medications, called Atypical Anti-psychotics, although having less of those problems, can cause significant weight gain and precipitate diabetes. Suffice it to say that, taken long-term, they can be very invasive, although worth the risk if the alternative is suffering from the ravages of Mania or Schizophrenia (discussed in Chapters 9 and 10). But used in small doses and for the short term (weeks, not months), either *Zyprexa* (generic: olanzepine) or *Seroquel* (generic: quetiapine), can be safe and effective medications to strategically add on to the others to help bring panic states under control.

BusPar (generic: buspirone) has been in the "corners" of psychiatry for several decades and was originally approved as a non addictive anti-anxiety medication. The problem I have found is that no one is really sure (including any of my patients) whether it works or not. Some feel that it is helpful as an adjunctive treatment along with antidepressants for the anxiety component of depression.

PHOBIAS

Panic represents the feedback reverberation of the two basic anxieties: separation anxiety and the anxiety in response to being trapped. Phobias occur when one or both of these two anxieties approach panic level in response to a specific experience such as being in open places (Agoraphobia) or closed in spaces (Claustrophobia). In both of these circumstances, the designation of phobic pathology is predicated on the degree to which the patient's behavior is dominated by defense against either separation anxiety or trapped anxiety devolving into panic. In such cases, a behavioral therapist who is skilled in desensitization techniques (read description of Behavior Therapy above) should take the lead with the psychiatrist in a consultant role. This advice also pertains to patients with excessive anxiety in social situations (Social Phobia), for whom the section on Chronicity at the end of Chapter 4 should be particularly be heeded because social phobia often results in unhealthy isolation if it persists over long periods of time.

When phobias occur only infrequently, the least invasive treatment is to attempt to anticipate the circumstance in which the anxiety will be triggered and "pre-medicate" with a low dose of a short acting benzodiazepine, such as lorazepam or alprazolam about an hour before the "event." If the phobic reactions are above a certain frequency, adding an SSRI either with or without the "targeted" use of benzodiazepines may be indicated. I must stress again that the principal treatment of phobias should be conducted by a therapist trained in desensitization techniques.

Low doses of the beta blocker, propranolol, have been used for public speaking or performance phobias for many years. Beta blockers block the effects of anxiety in the periphery of the body at the junction between the nerves and muscles, so they help to lower heart rate and prevent hand tremors under those conditions. In severe cases, small doses of both propranolol and a short acting benzodiazepine may be prescribed. It goes without saying that these treatments should be tested at home first with monitoring of (slowing of the) pulse, (lowering of) blood pressure, and the occurrence of dizziness.

GENERALIZED ANXIETY DISORDER (GAD)

Generalized Anxiety Disorder by definition is chronic anxiety which is pathological but below Panic level. Both cognitive and insight oriented therapists view pathological anxiety as faulty emotional responses to the reality the patient's current circumstances. The cognitive therapist attempts to demonstrate to the patient the logical inconsistencies of their emotional responses, while the insight oriented therapist attempts to correspond patterns of the current emotional distortions with those in their childhood circumstances. Both therapies, by virtue of their continuing focus on the patient's anxiety problems, are constantly helping the patient through desensitization. Some patients are interested in delving into the depths of their emotional lives, while others simply are not. The latter, "2 and 2 equals 4" logical types are good candidates for cognitive therapy which is usually time-limited with "homework" assignments. In GAD, it is of particular importance to gently probe patient's childhood for anything unusual in order to help in deciding whether to advise the patient to undertake the commitment of open-ended years of Insight Oriented Therapy.

In any case, it is established wisdom in the field that an important ingredient to the success of any psychiatric therapy, including medication, is the degree to which the purveyor of the treatment believes that their particular method can and does work. Of course, it helps that both cognitive and medication therapies have been demonstrated to be effective by placebo controlled, blinded studies, but it is impossible to measure the placebo effect of the belief itself that is inspired by this science. I personally witnessed this effect when Prozac first hit the market in 1988. There were inflated beliefs (a huge green and white Prozac capsule was on the cover of Time Magazine) that this was finally the answer to everyone's problems. I feel confident that this enthusiasm contributed to some of the spectacular patient responses to Prozac common in that era but just not seen any more. There is no question in my mind that the SSRI's are effective for anxiety, but not like back in the late 80's and early 90's when Prozac packed a little bit of magic.

Although psychotherapy should be seriously considered in GAD, treatment with medications is also often indicated. The section on Chronicity should be read at the end of Chapter 4. Because the condition is chronic, medication treatments often need to be chronically administered. As a result, extra effort is be made to pursue treatment options with the antidepressants and to limit benzodiazepines to intermittent use. Occasionally, if the anxiety is unremitting despite vigorous antidepressant trials, maintenance treatment with benzodiazepines may be warranted.

ANXIETY: MENTAL ILLNESS OR GOD-GIVEN ATTRIBUTE

This section began with the entity of Panic because of its unimpeachable credentials as an illness which needs to be wrestled to the ground with whatever tools are available. I have expressed my conviction that the underlying dynamic producing panic is the release into uncontrolled feedback reverberation of the two basic human anxieties of being trapped and of being abandoned which cause phobias when attached to specific circumstances. The human species is distinguished in that individuals possess a wide variety of complementary temperaments that functionally fit together to form an interdependent community. When considering an individual's capacity for anxiety, it can be viewed as how the components of temperament are balanced within this or that individual, or as to how these same components are balanced within this or that society. Thus the spectrum of anxiety problems below the threshold of panic may be seen as either an imbalance within the individual or rather an imbalance within a society which devalues the functions for which anxiety was evolved.

I have noted in myself a slow transformation over the many years of busy practice from a young doctor aggressively exhorting change within my patients to, more recently, tending to preach the gospel of acceptance of who they have become. I suspect that my Presbyterian heritage is crystallizing in my addled brain. The people I see are stressed out. They feel economically trapped and squeezed. They feel alone, alienated, and worried sick about their children. I can not help myself from seeing them as too gentle and sensitive to live within what the world has become. It has been my experience that the many hours I have spent in the attempt to link generalized anxiety conditions to childhood interaction with patients' parents has not produced any symptomatic relief unless these interactions were clearly abusive and traumatic (see chapter on Post-Traumatic Stress Disorder). I have watched through the years the meaning of my patients' anxieties migrate out from them and their families and into an environment over which they have limited control.

I remind myself that I am just a humble doctor whose simple mission is to alleviate the suffering in the patients in front of me. I attempt to extricate them from the belief that they are losers in a social game and to dignify their suffering as real. I gently try to point out to them that their lives are, indeed, a trap, and that they are, indeed, enmeshed within relationships where separation is a real component. I try to convince them that the reason that they suffer is that they are more sensitive to these realities of life. With notable exceptions, my patients have not been interested in disrupting the lives that they have built.

Generally I have found my role as therapist has become to gently nudge my patients back into their lives, and, with the added clarity of their specific sensitivity to being trapped or abandoned, to help them desensitize their anxieties to those elements in their lives that, together, we agree are inevitable. I exhort the discipline of relaxation, exercise, meditation, and yoga, and, yes, I give drugs, mainly antidepressants in as low a dose as I can get away with. I am as clear as I can be as to the Faustian[5] nature of this act of "dumbing down" my patient's emotional sensitivities in order for them to better fit into their Procrustean[6] lives. I make the judgment that their anxiety is more of a threat to their health than the long term side effects of these pills. You see my discomfort in the difficulties of sorting out my role as doctor with these anxious patients, and will hopefully understand my natural tendency to veer back into the discussion of conditions that can be more clearly defined as illnesses.

---

[5] Faust is a fictional figure who made a pact with the devil.
[6] Procrustes was a mythical Greek giant who stretched or shortened his captives to make them fit his beds.

HYSTERIA AND SUICIDE

Hysteria is a psychiatric symptom noted by Hippocrates to whose solemn oath all young doctors pledge themselves. The concept has always been controversial for many reasons, including being used as a sexist label, and as a term of stigma for psychiatric patients in general. Perhaps it should be thrown into the verbal dustbin along with neurosis, but I can think of no alternative.

Hysteria is an interactional dimension of anxiety. I previously used hysteria as an example of feedback reverberation resulting from the contagion of fear between two or more people. Psychiatric hysteria within a patient is different, although both separation anxiety and its kissing cousin, hysteria, are entities that also dwell within the social sphere. The reverberating circuit of hysteria does not exist exclusively within the patient, but also within the relational network of people around the patient. On a very general level hysteria is an incremental embellishment of anxious behavior serving to beseech a caretaking reaction from others. Intrinsic to hysteria is an underlying demanding tone which automatically triggers negative reactions in others springing from their sensitivity to being "trapped" by it. The sufferer of hysteria is equally attuned and tuned up by this implied rejection, escalating the intensity in a dangerous, vicious cycle, the end game of which can be a dangerous suicide gesture. It is a fundamental discipline which is required of those who treat mental illness to develop an acute awareness of and to control one's negative responses to hysteria in a patient.

The best advice is always try to remain as un-anxious as possible; try to cool things down by listening and controlling reflexive irritation. When talking to a patient who is hysterical, try not to react to the emotional "static" but rather attempt to intently focus on the content of what is being said in order to determine whether he or she has thought about suicide. If there is even a hint of yes, then that becomes the central issue. If the patient leaves the door open even slightly as to the possibility of suicide, get out front with very strong advice to seek admission to the psychiatric unit in a hospital. This is not a time to worry about the niceties of confidentiality. Start alerting relatives on the spot with the patient listening in front of you. Do not take no for an answer. As I used to tell medical students, "Do not wait until the train leaves the station; be waiting at the station when it arrives."

If a child is threatening suicide, and is resisting getting help, have the family take him or her to a hospital; if a suicidal adult is resisting, call the police. The message is: everything is negotiable except suicide. If suicide is left as an open possibility, the only alternative to hospitalization is constant monitoring by responsible family members. In calmly raising the stakes by the insistence upon effective actions in response to the face value of what is being said, you penetrate the hysteria by directly addressing its basic request to be meaningfully cared for. But, then again, flexibility is always useful in such incendiary circumstances. If you feel the grip of hysteria is relaxing, sit back and give the patient the opportunity to convince you that he or she has taken back control of his or her emotions.

HYSTERICAL "OVERLAY" IN SICKNESS AND "UNDERLIE" IN MARRIAGE

Temperament is the part of the person's behavior which is inherited genetically. Personality is the end product of the interaction between temperament and environmental experience. Freud made much of an arrested infantile sexuality in hysteria whereas I see genetically high separation sensitivity having been over sensitized and "stuck" in childhood. Either way, anxiety in hysteria is specifically relieved by the care of parental figures and is exacerbated if this care is rejected.

For the patient with hysteria, non psychiatric sickness can become a vehicle whereby sanctuary is sought through the ministrations of a physician. Similar in kind to the above approach to the patient threatening suicide, the physician must resist negative responses to hysterical "overlay" which exaggerate the symptoms of an illness. One's irritation toward this phenomenon can be constrained and transformed into a diagnostic instrument which informs the presence of a second condition while treating the underlying substrate of the first.

Much of psychiatry is in the timing; in this case having the patience to wait for and then to seize the right moment to strongly recommend commitment to Insight Oriented Psychotherapy. I have seen these patients improve with the insight that the hysterical behavior is an expression of underlying separation anxiety and fear of abandonment carried out from childhood, which then can be faced squarely and desensitized with the help of a persistent therapist.

In addition, hysteria is often locked into the underside of marital relationships. The classic situation is that the person who is most fearful of separation "traps" the other with his or her fearful anger, whereupon the person who is trapped "goes underground" with his or her own resentment, which can slowly transform into a bilious distain and start leaking out like poison. If you point a gun at your wife and demand that she love you, she will say, "Of course, my dear!" But does she really mean it? Hysteria is not just the demanding scream for love; it is also its quarry secretly simmering in response. Symptoms arising from this endemic parasite in relationships can flare up to produce florid forms of Atypical Depression, as shall be mentioned in the following Chapter, but effective treatment in these difficult cases must include both parties.

Chapter 4

PATHOLOGICAL DEPRESSION: THE SHUTDOWN RESPONSE

Upon occasion, I have been called in to consult on a patient who has sustained a significant physical sickness, particularly prolonged infection, because the relatives are alarmed at the concurrent depression in the patient. Most often these symptoms do not consist of active negative or suicidal thinking, but, rather, lack of emotional initiative or responsiveness. I have explained to the relatives that this is a natural reaction of the brain to the sickness, most probably to conserve the body's energy to fight the disease, and that normal emotional behavior will reliably return when the underlying illness resolves. I have become convinced by my patient's descriptions of depression that a significant component of it is similarly a reactive shutdown of the brain in response to the pathological intensity of specifically painful kinds of anxiety. In effect, the shutdown response is a backup defense which kicks in to control the hyperactivity of feedback reverberation when negative feedback controls fail. As a result, depression is experienced as a confusing combination of intensely painful anxiety along side shutdown symptoms of lack of initiative and will power.

ATYPICAL DEPRESSION: SEPARATION ANXIETY

As a quirk of history, the special category of depression caused by separation anxiety, even though it is the most common kind of depression, is officially called Atypical Depression. When describing depression, I like to start with Atypical Depression because the dynamic and reactive nature of the depressive shutdown response is most clearly revealed. It was by carefully listening to the emotional fluctuations in reaction to the vicissitudes of the separation scenarios driving this process that I first realized that a significant component of depression functions as an emergency shutdown switch on emotions when they are spinning too fast. These patients can precisely articulate about the shutdown symptoms kicking in at a certain level of intensity in their obsessive, internal struggle, but then, suddenly kick back out in direct response to this feedback reverberation ceasing when hope is ignited by some positive contact occurring within a tenuous, romantic relationship.

It would seem that when negative feedback controls fail and feedback reverberation takes over, there is a "backup" shutdown switch which is tripped. The shutdown symptoms are the brain's reactive defense against the malignantly painful hyperactivity of the illness itself, in the same way a fever is a reactive defense against an infection. Perhaps the shutdown response decreases the incidence of suicide. It is a well known phenomenon in the treatment of depression that if the shutdown symptoms lift before the feedback reverberation, there is an increased risk for suicide.

The intensity with which a person emotionally reacts to the rupture of a close interpersonal relationship is a fundamental aspect of who that person is. Among others, one emotional underpinning of a loyal, committed friend who really cares about you is separation anxiety. All and all, probably the majority of the office consultations I have seen over the years have been the trials and tribulations of people who, whether caused by genes or experience, have ended up in life with high sensitivities to separation. Randomly turn on some country music on the radio and there is a good chance the subject concerns the pain of being dumped by a girl or boy friend. You might say, "Get over it."

This is a good place to introduce a peculiar paradox. Patients who become mentally ill in circumstances that others can easily identify as difficult are often not given psychiatric treatment because people think to themselves, "If I were in that situation (dying of cancer, death of a spouse, dumped by a boy or girl friend, or even being very old), I would feel terrible too." These are situations in which it is important to differentiate existential blues from illness (a squeal in the P.A. system).

The initial negotiation phase of a romantic relationship is the toughest time of life for a person burdened with excessive separation anxiety. Crash course on relationships: Who is afraid of being trapped, and who is afraid of being left? If the gap is too wide, the first one takes a step back, the second one lunges forward, which further entraps the first, who then dumps the second. If you are endowed with a high sensitivity to separation, in the politics (we are now talking about power, which has the tendency to corrupt) of romantic relations, you will always end up the loser. Although everyone can relate to being dumped by a girl or boyfriend, this kind of circumstance can cause some unfortunate people to become mentally ill, which may last months or even years. Mental illness is determined by a sustained level of emotional intensity completely dominating the mind. In people who are vulnerable, the intensity of separation anxiety increases exponentially as they become more romantically involved. The other person who is the object of this intensity might not be able to hide feeling trapped by it, which then further escalates the back and forth of separation anxiety in response to more feelings of being trapped in a familiar vicious cycle, sometimes ending with an exquisitely painful condition that can amply qualify as a mental illness.

This condition is characterized by severe, unremitting, painful anxiety, which is very much focused on the loss of the love relationship. To repeat, all mental illness is the loss of control in the modulation of emotional entities interacting with each other in a feedback manner such that they "squeal" into hyper-intensity. In the illness of Panic, separation anxiety enters into feedback reverberation with the anxiety of being trapped. In this case separation anxiety is thrown into a high pitch in response to a lost relationship, but then transforms into a rapidly oscillating response to the memories of the love lost. The mind of the patient is dominated by separation anxiety, which compels the patient into memories of the lost closeness. The intensity of depressive anxiety is driven into illness by the relentless "yo-yo" of internal switching between memories of past intimacy and the reality that it no longer exists. Separation anxiety internally driven to such a high pitch has a specifically tragic tonality to it in the direction of feeling worthless and abandoned. Crying and the feelings of sadness behind it serve as signals to family and friends to rally around and are central characteristics of the underlying intensity of depression but one additional component defines it as medically clinical depression.

This internalized oscillation of separation anxiety at a variable threshold of intensity shuts down the patient's emotional system in a characteristic way, with which it is impossible to truly empathize because it is not within the realm of normal experience. It is this shutdown response that is an intrinsic component of the phenomenon of clinical depression. I have prodded thousands of depressed patients to help me in my attempt to describe it. The main difficulty here is to distinguish between simple tiredness or fatigue and what I have come to understand as the most central aspect of depression: the evaporation of the will to do anything. All initiative to do ordinary, routine tasks in your life disappears. Upon awakening in the morning one realizes with dismay that it is going to take a monumental act of will to get up and brush one's teeth, let alone get dressed and go to work. Normal motivation has been "unplugged" such that one has to drag oneself through the day.

The painful "yo-yoing" starts on the outside, in the relationship, but then transposes itself inside the patient's mind where it spins up into illness triggering the compensatory shutdown response. Often these patients are having a hard time restraining themselves from unwisely calling up the lost person, even after they have been roundly rejected, just for the momentary relief afforded by a brief contact even though the inevitable further rejection makes it worse. As stated, a similar dynamic occurs within the patient's own mind. Because the feeling of being separated from the person is so painful, their mind automatically finds relief by hiding in memories of being close, but then reeling back and forth, in and out of reality.

I have focused on the circumstance of rejection in the context of love lost because of the frequency of its occurrence and because the vicissitudes of an on and off relationship first clearly revealed to me both the specific nature of the internal emotional feedback reverberation and that the shutdown response was reactive to it. However, Atypical Depression can occur in other situations, such as children leaving for camp or college, and, most notably forms the core dynamic in a grief reaction to the death of a family member which ranges from normal to severe forms of pathological grief. Pathological grief is a particularly malignant form of Atypical Depression in which suicide often assumes the form of joining the deceased person.

TREATMENT OF ATYPICAL DEPRESSION

I point out to patients suffering from Atypical Depression that it is the process and not the fact of separation that is so painful. It is the actual emotional movement from being close to not being close that hurts so much. Once that movement stops and one has installed oneself at a certain distance from the person, the pain remits. Recall the Law of Desensitization in Behavioral Therapy, described in Chapter 4, which states that avoiding the object of anxiety makes it worse, and a measured exposure to it eventually resolves it. The patient with Atypical Depression is hiding, and avoiding the pain of being separated by existing momentarily, back and forth, within a dream world of memories, and, therefore the anxiety gets worse.

So part of therapy has to be slow exposure to the separation anxiety intrinsic to the loss, and, following the Law of Desensitization, it will remit with time. The kinds of advice for people facing emotional rejection includes telling a wife who is pushing away her husband through desperately holding on that "the only way to have him is to let him go"; or telling the unrequited dumpee who is refusing to let go of a hopeless relationship that "Even if the sole and only goal of this advice was to get her back, it would be the same: Let her go," and then adding gratuitously, "Your grandmother could have given you the same advice."

One can see the same general issues in the process of grief for deceased family members in that the retention of vivid memories of the deceased person's suffering, as painful as they are, is less painful than that of letting them go. To the extent that these conditions have not crossed the threshold of illness with activation of a shutdown response and, therefore, are tractable to psychotherapy, the therapist must be less the surgeon and more the obstetrician, slowly guiding the delivery of these patients back to themselves.

MEDICATIONS IN THE TREATMENT OF ATYPICAL DEPRESSION

As an introduction to both sections describing the treatment of depression with antidepressants, it is important for the patient to be aware that antidepressants rarely can precipitate subtle forms of mania. For this reason, it is important to read the section on "Mixed State Bipolar Disorder" in Chapter 9.

An otherwise healthy patient presenting in the office distraught about a current relationship with a history of many similarly traumatic breakups certainly is a candidate for either Cognitive or Insight Oriented Psychotherapy. However, I feel strongly that there is an underutilized role for medication in these cases. Often, even small doses of an SSRI can substantially and promptly decrease the separation anxiety in acute cases of interpersonal rejection. The experience of taking a medication and feeling relief from this kind of interpersonal stress can be very therapeutic in that it illustrates the degree to which their problem stems from a simple hypersensitivity to separation. Some of these patients have benefited by prophylacticaly taking small doses of an SSRI as they enter into a new relationship finding that they can better maintain their stability due to the increased modulation of their separation anxiety.

Atypical Depression can be severe and its treatment, like in other kinds of depression, is not always easy. Sometimes patients simply do not tolerate the medications or do not respond after many trials. To summarize, in a patient with prolonged depression, the designation of the diagnosis-type as being Atypical means that: 1) Separation sensitivity has played a decisive role in the genesis of the depression. 2) the patient has high anxiety and 3) the patient has marked "shutdown" symptoms. The most characteristic feature is that separation sensitivity is either ongoing as a mental dynamic or was the original precipitant. My impression is that in Atypical Depression, as with other forms of depression, the longer these conditions last, the more entrenched the shutdown symptoms become. No longer a simple brain response to anxiety, these two components seem to metastasize into each other to become inseparable mixtures of anxiety and empty enervation overlain with a reactive sense of hopelessness, helplessness, and self-loathing.

For these entrenched cases, it is generally felt that, in addition to the SSRI's, medications with a more stimulating effect, such as those which increase brain levels of either norepinephrine or even dopamine are needed. Strategies include adding *Wellbutrin* (available as buprobion) to an SSRI. Another good option is switching to *Cymbalta* (generic: duloxetine) or *Effexor XR* (available as venlafaxin XR), even up to high doses. At some point in the treatment of severe, intractable Atypical Depression, the monoamine oxidase inhibitors (MAOI's): either

Nardil or *Parnate* might be considered. The MAOI's were the first class of antidepressant discovered in the 1950s,[7] and remain the most powerful drugs, particularly for the treatment of severe, treatment-resistant Atypical Depression. Taking MAOIs is fraught with many problems. First, they are incompatible with all other antidepressants, which need to be stopped for at least two weeks before they are started (the same pertains after stopping an MAOI and starting another antidepressant). They are potentially very dangerous because they interact with the amino acid tyramine, mainly found in preserved meats and aged cheeses, (Deli-pizza-type food) and "heavy" red wines such as Chianti. Also, cold medicines containing ephedrine-type components, and *Demerol* are contraindicated. A more complete list should be given to the patient. If patients accidentally ingest one of these common foods or drugs, they are at high risk for a hypertensive crisis, producing a pounding headache, and there exists the possibility of cerebral hemorrhage. The patient's diet therefore becomes somewhat of a mine field fraught with a potentially fatal reaction. I have had many patients whose suffering led them to assume these risks after careful consideration, even though chances of successful responses to antidepressants generally decrease with each succeeding trial. Electroconvulsive treatment (which will be discussed later) is also an option if nothing else works.

The cautionary note introduced in the section on hysteria shall be repeated. If the patient with Atypical Depression is married or in a binding relationship, one must consider whether the condition is a result of a separation-rejection process of

---

[7] The original MAOI was synthesized from leftover WWII German V2 rocket fuel!

hysteria (see section at the end of Chapter 3) that covertly lies within the relationship, even though the symptoms are in the patient. It is important to note that the couple is often unaware that their interaction is causing the psychiatric symptoms. These situations can be extremely destructive to whole families, and the symptoms produced can be very complex, changeable, and of great intensity. Often, the "proof of the pudding" only emerges after the couple tumultuously separates, whereupon the patient simply recovers.

In retrospect, that one can see that the pathology existed within the relationship. The needy, separation-sensitive patient crosses a "feeling trapped" threshold in the spouse, which has the effect of the spouse's withdrawal of affection, which in turn sets off more separation anxiety, causing more trapped feelings in the spouse in a vicious cycle that can become instantiated in an unhappy marriage. This emotional cancer can surely manifest as mental illness, with enigmatic, shifting and florid presentations. Although relational elements are usually clear enough, the alarming psychiatric symptoms in the patient afflicted with this nasty form of Atypical Depression can lure the psychiatrist into a headlong chasing of elusive symptoms with changing diagnoses, multiple drugs and even electroconvulsive treatments, all to no avail. Such cases are rare, but I feel they are commonly misunderstood.

MELANCHOLIC DEPRESSION: THE FEAR OF BEING TRAPPED

Many patients who have suffered severe Melancholic Depression argue persuasively that it is the most painful of human afflictions. Aptly named by Hippocrates, melancholia means "black bile" because for sufferers, it is as if the soul has been supplanted by a bitter, inky substance. In the preceding discussion, the general subjective feature of mental illness has been described as emotional entities locking together into the hyperactivity of a reverberating circuit. In panic, the fear of being trapped locks up with the fear of separation within a single mind, and in hysteria, these two fears do so across relationships. In Atypical Depression, the fear of separation locks up into feedback reverberation in response to memories of a lost relationship, which then triggers the "shutdown" response characteristic of depression.

The most established animal model for depression has been to place a rodent in a glass cylinder which is half full of water. The animal struggles for a while to get out but cannot due to the slickness of the glass sides. After a variable amount of time, the animal floats back passively. Antidepressants increase the time that the animal struggles before the occurrence of this shutdown response such that it is an excellent predictor of antidepressant response in humans.

In Melancholic Depression, the fear of being trapped (trapped anxiety) increases to a threshold that then triggers this same shutdown response. In Atypical Depression, the shutdown response does not directly affect the basic illness, which is comprised of separation anxiety interacting with loss. In stark contrast, in Melancholia, the shutdown response strikes the fear of being trapped directly between the eyes. The result is that the fear of being trapped locks up in interaction with the shutdown response itself; each element stimulates the other in a virulent and malignant example of feedback reverberation.

In general, the fear of being trapped exists not just within relationships, but as an underlying general motivation. In everyday life, an emotional "push" is afforded by the avoidance of anxiety that arises from the feeling of being trapped by the confines that life inevitably imposes. Economists refer to fear and greed in the marketplace. The fear to which they refer is ultimately the trap of poverty. The ordinary person, in different measures, is thusly pushed into the performance of deeds and work and generally making one's way out of the confines imposed by the circumstances in which one finds oneself. Such an orientation, far from a sickness, goes to the very heart of the life impulse itself. Indeed, the central ethos that binds us as a nation is the idea of freedom, the business of which is the constant striving to extract ourselves not just the from the trap of poverty but that of tyranny in all its varied forms.

Whereas those on the sensitive end of a spectrum of separation sensitivity sacrifice their freedom in order to maintain personal connections, those on the sensitive end of a spectrum of trap sensitivity tend to do the opposite. This sensitivity is particularly attuned to fluxes in the politics of life. Similar to separation sensitivity, it is sudden change that triggers illness. An economic reversal, a perceived loss of status, the discovery of an illness, or the natural decline produced by advancing age may herald Melancholia. This sickness lies in the failure of control of the very fear of being trapped as one feels oneself slipping back as into a deep and desperate hole.

The drug curare, when injected, causes the paralysis of all voluntary muscles by blocking transmission at the neuromuscular junction. Derivatives of curare are used in surgery to obtain relaxation of the muscles and are also part of most protocols for execution by lethal injection. Contemplate for a moment how it would feel to be injected with curare and suddenly lose command of all your muscles. Perhaps the better comparison to how Melancholia feels is to imagine this happening from the point of view of your body suddenly losing its central command.

At a certain threshold of anxiety, the same shutdown reaction as is found in Atypical Depression occurs with a failure of all motivation as described above, but, in Melancholia, it is this very failure that stimulates the further fear of being trapped, which, in turn, renders even more paralysis. All the fears that are daily quenched by the esteem of productive work and of fitting into the scheme of things are exaggerated beyond imagination with both frightful flogging of the self and dreadful feelings of being cast into oblivion. Not uncommonly, in those so predisposed, protracted and intense convictions of guilt, the feeling that one has caused and is causing other people's suffering, predominates.

In talking to patients with Melancholia, you have to deal with the self-fulfilling prophesy of their predicament. They are actually unable to function, which does cause problems in their lives, but there is no mental illness in which it is more important to staunchly uphold the medical model that the problem truly is a sickness. Their assertions that "life is over" and "not worth living" must be met with fervent assertions that such beliefs are themselves the afflictions of a powerful disease which can and should be aggressively treated by a psychiatrist. Thoughts and impulses to commit suicide characteristically do not have an hysterical overlay, but are rather an expression, intrinsic to the condition, of the impulse to escape this intolerable entrapment; So all the more so, the response to talk of suicide should be strongly the same as discussed above in the section on Hysteria and Suicide in Chapter 3.

The professional judgment will be made as to whether the patient is too sick to work, and, if so, what to tell the workplace. Owing to the persisting reality of stigma, I sometimes have counseled patients to report that their doctor has ordered them not to work while leaving the details of the condition vague: "He's not sure of the diagnosis." Privacy concerning the details of an illness is the patient's sacred right and should be defended stoutly. On the other hand, the patient may trust an enlightened supervisor to use this information in the best interest of the patient. The patient may be told not to engage in activities that are centrally disabled by the condition from which they suffer, such as those demanding the extended maintenance of concentration or complex, interpersonal interactions. "Mindless" activities, in order to divert and engage the mind, such as walking, gardening, light housework or easy reading, are often recommended.

Certain factors increase the risks of suicide in patients afflicted with Melancholia. Alcohol consumption, whether or not the patient is deemed "an alcoholic," should be stopped, at least initially, in all cases of severe mental illness, but particularly in Melancholia. Reliable information must be obtained on this issue either way, because, if the patient is accustomed to significant drinking, even mild withdrawal could suddenly exacerbate the condition without the support of benzodiazepine tranquilizers. Problems associated with alcohol, and addiction in general, will be thoroughly covered in Chapter 8.

Another, somewhat paradoxical risk is the pre-existing temperament of the patient. The somewhat over-responsible, guilt-driven person is a classic case, but the hard-charging, "Type A" personalities who are in positions of leadership can particularly become suicidal when afflicted with Melancholia. It seems that the same drive, which in health was directed "outward and upward," is, in a virulent reaction to the shutdown symptoms, cruelly and with savage intensity, twisted around and aimed back "in and down" upon themselves (drive reversal). A patient suffering from Atypical Depression in a state of pathological grief may think about committing suicide to join the deceased. In contrast, the patient with Melancholia is driven to suicide as an escape not only from the excruciating pain, but also because it is the very hypersensitivity to being trapped within these patients which is unbearably amplified by the illness. The image of the impulse to leap out from the World Trade Center comes to mind. And then, lastly, if a separation or divorce, with added features of Atypical Depression is heaped on top, the risk of suicide increases greatly.

In crisis situations, difficult questions must be asked, such as whether the patient has thought through a method of suicide. Firearms should be taken from the house. When dealing with the actual occurrence of suicide in severe Melancholia, it is important for relatives and friends and, indeed, the doctor and therapist, to maintain perspective. The other side of the stigma of mental illness is that, because it is "all in your head," it would seem to follow that it should be able to be controlled by, say, just talking them out of it. Although the good doctor should always be the purveyor of eternal hope with endless further treatments and expert consultations, in the retrospection of a suicide, Melancholia can sometimes be viewed as the equivalent of a malignant cancer in the brain.

TREATMENT OF MELANCHOLIC DEPRESSION

Acute Melancholic Depression is harder to treat than Atypical Depression because of its more completely self contained nature. The "drive reversal" phenomenon described above can cause fixed delusional beliefs that everything is beyond repair and hopeless. It is well to have a therapist schooled in Cognitive Therapy to gently, but relentlessly pound away at the flaws in these beliefs. In order to counteract a tendency for friends and family to be "brain washed" by the illness, I feel it is appropriate for them to ask the patient to ask the therapist to invite them to attend these sessions on occasion so they can watch the application of logic by an expert.

Admission to the psychiatric unit of a hospital can be therapeutic in and of itself, not only for the release of care into the protective hands of professionals but also to reinforce the status of patienthood. Sometimes desensitization to the comfortable and secure "trap" of being confined to a hospital can by proxy relax the internal dynamic of being trapped by the illness. A halfway measure in this direction, which is often recommended, is admission into a day hospital in which the patient participates in therapeutic group activities and active medication management during the day, but remains at home at night.

The psychiatrist's main weapons are an arsenal of physical treatments, mainly drugs, but also available is electroconvulsive treatment. It is common for the psychiatrist to take the lead when the symptoms are acute and these treatments are in flux, and then to drop into the background when things have stabilized while the therapist consolidates the gains. Often it is well for the spouse (and family) to be involved in therapy in order to sort out the disruption of suddenly having been thrown into a relationship of caretaker to the patient and then to readjust into the pre-existing partnership.

MEDICATIONS IN MELANCHOLIA

As an introduction to both sections describing the treatment of depression with antidepressants, it is important for the patient to be aware that rarely, antidepressants can precipitate subtle forms of mania. For this reason, it is important to read the section on "Mixed State Bipolar Disorder" in Chapter 9.

The full range of medication treatment for Melancholic Depression exceeds the scope of this writing, and there is no single approach that has been scientifically proven to be the most effective. The basic idea is similar to that in the treatment of Atypical Depression described above, but, commonly, goes well beyond. There is always a tension between the need to be aggressive and move onto "bigger" treatments, and the need for patience, to wait for more time sufficient for existing treatments to kick in and work. There are four classes of antidepressants: the SSRI's and monoamine oxidase inhibitors or MAOI's, both of which were mentioned above; the tricyclic antidepressants, used before Prozac, and then the newer, combination drugs with serotonin and nor-epinephrine effects (sometimes called SNRI's), such as Effexor XR (available as venlafaxin XR), and, the newest, Cymbalta (generic: duloxetine). Also, there is Wellbutrin SR (available as bupropion SR), which is in a class by itself. The overall rule is to start with treatments with less side effects and risks, and to slowly and deliberately allow the strength of the symptoms to dictate stronger treatments with the possibility of more negative side effects.

There are two tracks of treatment: one is the core treatment with one, or even a combination, of the above mentioned antidepressants, and the second is to add adjunctive medicines. A common progression of the core treatment would be to start with an SSRI antidepressant; then push the dose to high levels, all the time keeping a running quantification of whether the symptoms are better, worse, or the same. A common next switch of the core antidepressant might be to *Cymbalta* (generic: duloxetine) or *Effexor XR* (available as venlafaxin XR). Concurrent to the core switching of antidepressants, adjunctive medications can be added. Adding a medication is a little easier because switching the antidepressants can be time consuming and disruptive. A common, time-honored adjunctive strategy is to add lithium to an established antidepressant regimen for 3-4 weeks. The addition of lithium occasionally boosts the effectiveness of the antidepressant to which it is added. However, usually the adjunctive medication which is added to the core antidepressant is targeted to a specific symptom such as agitation, anxiety, or lack of energy.

A distinction is made between agitation and anxiety. Agitation has a physical aspect to it, almost like the whole body is in a state of tightly held tremor, whereas anxiety is constant mental fear. Introducing doses of a benzodiazepine tranquilizer for anxiety, and small doses of an Atypical Antipsychotic, either Zyprexa (generic: olanzepine) or Seroquel (generic: quetiapine) for agitation is common with appropriate warnings about side effects, which are fully considered in the section in Chapter 10 on the treatment of Schizophrenia. If lethargy and lack of energy are present, options include adding Wellbutrin SR (available as bupropion SR) to an established antidepressant, or, alternatively, adding Provigil (generic: modafinil - approved for narcolepsy), or even stimulants like Ritalin (available as methylphenidate) and Dexedrine (available as dextroamphetamine). In addition, the patient may need sleeping pills for proper sleep.

If none of this is working, and months have gone by while the patient continues to suffer, consultation with a specialist in treatment-resistant depression is often warranted. There are wide varieties of drug treatment strategies available and, beyond a level of complexity; I have always felt more comfortable proceeding with the guidance of such a specialist.

ELECTROCONVULSIVE TREATMENT (ECT)

ECT is thought to be the most effective treatment for treatment-resistant depression of all varieties. The decision as to whether to resort to electroconvulsive treatment should be a family decision, guided by a specialist in the field. The most consistent side effect of ECT is mental confusion, as will be described, but, when first contemplating this treatment, it must be acknowledged that the very idea of inducing an epileptic convulsion via electrocution, albeit carefully controlled, is, indeed, shocking. All the Frankenstein images of the power-hungry doctor manipulating the helpless patient attach themselves to ECT.

In ECT, a seizure is induced by delivering an electric current to the brain. The exact mechanism of how this helps depression is controversial. The following school of thought makes sense to me. The massive stimulation of the seizure causes compensatory post seizure (post-ictal) inhibition of the underlying pathological hyperactive feedback reverberation causing the re-establishment of its modulation and regulation, at least for a period of weeks. A gross analogy would be, if the engine in your car was racing, you might gun the motor a couple of times to un-stick mechanical negative feedback mechanisms in the carburetor which then return the engine to its normal idle.

The procedure itself is very safe. A short-acting general anesthetic is injected, followed by a curare-type medication which paralyzes all the muscles such that, when the electrodes are placed on the head and the current delivered, virtually no movement is observed during the ensuing seizure. Meanwhile an anesthesiologist breathes for the patient and vital signs are monitored closely. The procedure may take 10-15 minutes, and then, upon awakening, there might follow the side-effects of the anesthesia, such as some nausea and headaches and lingering grogginess. ECT is commonly done as an out-patient, with a caretaker (alternatively husband /wife /son /daughter) driving and staying with the patient during the intensive course and for several weeks afterwards, until the confusion clears. Sometimes at the peak of confusion, it is well that the patient be in the hospital where the treatments are administered.

Some disorientation is expected to appear in a week after roughly 3 treatments. A standard course of treatment is 8 given 3 times per week for 2 ½ weeks. Mainly due to this confusion,[8] the patient needs 24 hour care until the confusion lifts, normally about 10 days after the final treatment. Honest controversy

---

[8] Curiously, the confusion is usually not bothersome to the patient, probably because of simultaneous improvement in the depression, although the confusion does not cause the improvement in mood. After recovery from both depression and ECT, usually there is a loss of memory not only for the weeks of intensive treatment, but also for the month or two prior to it, an aspect which, often, friends and family feel is positive.

continues to surround the issue of residual decrease in memory function for months or even years after the treatments. Suffice it to say that this possibility should be considered when making the initial decision. The other issue is how long the improvement rendered by a course of ECT will last. This is a common issue, and seasoned judgment needs to be exercised as to whether the re-establishment of prophylactic medications is sufficient, or whether there is continuing need to administer ECT once a week, decreasing, perhaps, to once a month, and ending when the patient's condition is clearly stable. ECT has long been a whipping boy for the anti-psychiatry movement. It is hard for me to believe that anyone could sustain such enmity if they had witnessed close at hand the stark, relentless brutality which Melancholia wreaks upon its victims.

CHRONICITY (AS IN CHRONIC)

It has often occurred to me that, in this new day of increasingly effective treatments, that patients suffering from the acute onset of the disruptive mental agony of mental illness are more likely to seek treatment due to its contrast with their prior state of health. However, some patients have had smoldering, lifelong, but, nevertheless pathological levels of anxiety (Generalized Anxiety Disorder) or depression (Dysthymic Disorder), "as long as I can remember." "I've never known anything else." These are the people who came out of the woodwork after Prozac became available after 1988, saying, "Oh! This is how everyone else feels." These are patients that the primary care physician should be on the lookout for and many can be well treated without significant complexity. I can assure you from written testimony of letters sent to me from longstanding patients upon my retirement, that there are many who have had an experience akin to stepping outside the doctor's door and "throwing away the crutches." (Well, not exactly; it takes a little longer than that.) I cannot be happier to have been the purveyor of health for all those patients who had spent a lifetime considering themselves as "depressives" or accepting the interpersonal exploitation which often accompanies longstanding anxiety conditions. To all these patients, I have given the exhortation to keep it in their mind that the medication is a "tool, and not a crutch!"

Chapter 5

Pathological Anger: Stress, Frustration and Violence

Stress can mean any circumstance that produces anxiety, but, for the purposes of this discussion, I will narrow it down to the "trap" produced by time. If one is in a set of circumstances to which one has to react, the stressful part is that you have to do it NOW, or before a certain time. The Type A personality describes those driven by time pressure to achieve more and more, even when relaxing. Type A personalities are particularly sensitive to the anxiety produced by the trap of time and live with a chronic experience of a daily race to keep ahead of its relentless curve. While the Type A personality is pushed by the fundamental relief afforded by escaping this trap, he is also pulled and energized by the extension of his powers through the commandeering of others into furthering his achievements, as if gathering momentum along a railroad track. But when failure is encountered by these movers and shakers of the world, or someone gets in the way, the mental train wreck, called frustration, occurs. Frustration tolerance is a highly learned virtue, but surely has its genetic bases as well.

There are those who simmer along in chronically frustrated states struggling to control their tempers and some who are not able to contain their anger. There is strong evidence that chronic mental states of anger can cause cardiovascular problems. Although the Type A personality is specifically suited for success in the business world, when the Type A person loses his or her temper, he or she loses in the game. Chronic loss of temper can cause problems both at work and home, and, famously, is dangerous on the road. Therapy in groups has become a well known modality for anger management and is comprised of the indoctrination of acceptance of responsibility for the problem's consequences through the consistent application of behavioral self-regulation techniques.

SSRI antidepressants can definitely help a temper problem. Some conditions, in which the explosive rage produced is way out of proportion to the provocation of the circumstances, could be caused by an unusual type of seizure and should be evaluated by a neurologist. If the behavior is not part of a longstanding pattern and is of recent onset, it could be part of a manic condition, which is discussed in Chapter 10.

Of course, the largest mental health problem in the world is anger leading to violence, in which justice must precede medicine. Just as the cause of mental illness is not known, the cause of violence is unknown and a description of the various types of people who end up in the criminal justice system goes beyond the scope of this Guidebook. I started out my career working in a prison system in a quest to understand exactly how the forces that regulate and restrain a temper problem in, let us say a type A personality, can break down into violence. Nowhere is the dynamic duality of mind, in this case the balance between anger and fear, more palpable than in a prison population. In prison culture, there is a "negative economy" of fear: no one wants it and everyone is trying to push it into someone else by "getting over," an in-your-face version of "putting something over." The close up experience of the victim of violence becomes a sink into which a wad of frustration is stuffed by the perpetrator, which can progress into a malignantly compulsive addiction. That violence is the most fundamental and direct solution to frustration was clearly revealed to me. I was aghast with horror as if gaping at the ancient bones of reality.

The emotion of anger tends to dominate its own justification. Anger is an emotion that does not look inwards, but only outwards towards the person who is the target of it. That is simply how anger works.[9] The source of anger only reverts back to its owner in the legal context if social boundaries are crossed such as perpetration of acts of violence. Thus, in order for a person so afflicted to attain the status and privileges of being a patient, they must, themselves, strive to consider their own behavior as pathological. One accurate measure of the civility of a nation might be the quality of response to such self-rehabilitative efforts put forth by those in its criminal justice system. The study and treatments of violence is a vast area of mental health, which is also a subspecialty with a small cadre of dedicated practitioners and investigators.

---

[9] I am skeptical of the notion of depression as "anger turned inwards." The phenomenon of "drive reversal" in Melancholia, discussed above seems like such an example, but is really frustration released by the shutdown response. Self-directed anger in hysteria is really directed at someone else. Guilt is certainly a form of anger directed at the self, but its origin is not the self. Although clearly biologically rooted in the brain, I believe that guilt emanates from society. I plan to write another book to describe exactly how that works.

SNIT DISORDER AND ABUSE

Those suffering from Snit Disorder[10] are patients who respond to separation with anger rather than anxiety. All marital relationships have their ups and downs, even on a daily basis. As with Atypical Depression, the most sensitive times, are when the mood of the couple is close, and things are going particularly well. During those delicate moments, if there should be a perturbation in the seamlessness of intimacy, such as the expression of mild frustration, or some "button" is pushed and a temporary distance is created, a quantum of anger is triggered, which then creates more separation and more reflexive anger. In an instant, the patient is plunged into a tumultuous self-sustaining mood of anger which is restrained by the fear of separation. Although the smoldering snit is sustained by the separation it causes (feedback reverberation), the fear of separation also serves to contain the expression of the destructive rage. This smoldering snit may last for hours, days or even sometimes weeks. The patient is all too painfully aware of the emotional separation caused by the extravagant excesses of his or her angry mood, but is, nonetheless, locked into responding to that same separation with thoughts of revenge, divorce, abdication, etc. The patient in a snit is cast down into an internal rampart in the struggle to maintain the delicate balance of that which permits us to be civilized: the fear of abandonment which is the restraining force on the destructive power of rage.

It is in the more malignant of these moods, often fueled by alcohol, or by the interaction of two people precipitating these

---

[10] This is a category created by the author and will not be known as such by others.

moods in one another, that anger can get the upper hand and abuse is the result. Whether by violent actions, words, or any other means, abuse occurs when the restraining influence of abandonment and separation is breeched and the frustration of anger is forcefully thrust upon another with intent to hurt. Relief within the abuser is obtained by the discharge of psychic injury into the abused partner. The addictive nature of this primitive avenue of release of tension, along with the progressive alienation it produces, leads to the all too familiar cycle of abuse.

Prolonged exposure to abuse is a leading cause of Post-Traumatic Stress Disorder described in Chapter 7. Typically, if the snit breaks down into the overt expression of abuse, it is then followed by remorse and anxiety in response to the alienation thus produced. In other words, although overwhelmed with rage, the snit sufferer maintains contact with the restraining influence of a baseline of separation anxiety, which also vitally serves as the emotional footing upon which any insight rests. However, it is only with the strict and thorough understanding that all abuse must cease immediately, perhaps backed by the authority of law, that these situations can improve, and then only with the uttermost commitment and effort of a therapist with specific training and experience and with both parties engaged. In the absence of abuse, these angry mood states, here quaintly named (by me) as snits, can more clearly be identified as a bone fide illnesses with tractability to treatment.

This particular brand of illness has been kept in the shadows by its own signature of humiliation and despair. The patient sees him or herself as "acting like an idiot," and wanting to "go out into the garden and eat worms." However, the patient is ultimately powerless to control it. I felt compelled to create this category, exposing the stigmatic term, snit, to the light of day, because, when not vilified by the abusive behavior it can produce, this mainly male affliction is routinely ridiculed as childish, or dismissed by professionals as "narcissistic" or "controlling." Timing is everything when giving advice on sensitive subjects. The physician should counsel the family to wait for a receptive moment to talk to the patient, when things are going well and the mood upbeat. Again, dignify the condition as a medical entity from which he appears to be suffering and counsel the patient to get help. In treatment of Snit Disorder, a therapist should take the lead, with a primary care physician or psychiatrist as the adjunct consult.

TREATMENT OF SNIT DISORDER

If the patient has sufficient insight into the problem, it is helpful to have the wife or partner at least partially involved in the therapy. It is important for the therapist to have a frank discussion with both about unacceptable behavior in the snit mode: certainly physical violence, demeaning language and threatening divorce. Standard advice if abusive lines are crossed (short of violence, which should become a legal issue) is to have the abused partner leave the home on the spot and spend the night elsewhere. Zero tolerance for abuse is the first priority. It is also important to bring the abused partner into the patient's struggle to control his anger by attempting to become sensitive to "hot button" issues and developing a supportive attitude when the patient is enveloped inside a snit. The aim is to transform toxic distain by the abused partner into therapeutic respect for demonstrated effort and results on the part of the patient.

All drinking must stop. Family members should be explained how to cordon off the illness from the patient who attempts to take responsibility for it. My preferred approach to this problem is focused directly at the pathological behavior. The patient is encouraged to start taking measurements of frequency, duration, and intensity so progress can be demonstrated. The triggering events are investigated for their common elements. I advocate the well-known mentality which is part of many ancient Asian warrior traditions of constant vigilance and anticipation, which should be heightened during periods of closeness, which are times of vulnerability. This is the kind of problem which is more likely to occur when the mood of this closeness is suddenly snatched away unexpectedly. The law of desensitization (see section on Behavior Therapy in Chapter 4) can be fruitfully employed by the patient by the reconsideration of small "glitches" in the relationship as "therapeutic opportunities" to test one's control over a certain quantity of separation anxiety, which is then held steady and tolerated, preventing it from tumbling into a self-sustaining, toxic mood of anger.

Anticipation is the weapon for prevention, but then, after the poison has been secreted, and the patient is trapped within the mood, "damage control" measures should be taken by the patient. When enthralled in anger, the principal advice is to separate from the partner and "play for time." When engaged in an argument, it is difficult for the patient suffering from Snit Disorder to separate, sometimes following around the partner with angry rehashes. There should a prearranged agreement ("doctor's orders") that, once the snit sets in, both partners attempt to separate calmly with the implicit understanding that this action does not connote rejection, but, rather the patient is granted open-ended time to "work on it." The patient is then on his or her own to wait until the anger lifts. I give the following advice to desensitize to low levels of anger: "Live with a given level of anger with the knowledge that it will pass." Exercising, taking a drive, doing busy work, or practicing meditation are all useful activities while allowing the mood to "play itself out." Meanwhile the average durations of recent episodes are kept in mind with the knowledge that only gradual improvements are to be expected. Then, when the mood lifts, take up where you left off with the satisfaction that progress has been made.

Small doses of antidepressants can help significantly in buffering anger reactivity in this problem, which can be tapered off as the problem improves. In my experience, Insight Oriented Psychotherapy focused on childhood trauma or, conversely, lack of anger management guidance in childhood, is more useful after the symptoms are bought under control by behavioral types of treatment described above.

BORDERLINE PERSONALITY DISORDER

Psychiatry's struggle to define the Borderline condition is similar to that of the Supreme Court justice with the definition of pornography: "I know it when I see it." This is a condition that mainly manifests itself in the context of close family relationships, particularly marriages. Patients with Borderline Disorder can often function well, and can be successful in a structured work environment. The people afflicted with this condition are extremely sensitive to separation and rejection, but in contradistinction to patients afflicted with Atypical Depression, who react with anxiety, those with Borderline Disorder, like those with Snit Disorder, react to rejection with anger.

Another profitable comparison is with hysteria. Both conditions are characterized by emotionally painful reactions to the issue of separation that drives their respective sufferers into pathologically manipulative interpersonal behavior. In hysteria, anxiety drives manipulations by the patient of his or her own behavior through dramatic remonstrations the most serious of which are gestures of suicide. In the Borderline condition, reactive anger drives manipulations by the patient of his or her spouse or partner's behavior. In hysteria, there is never any question who the patient is, whereas the individual with Borderline Disorder often not only rejects but positively objects to the designation of patient.

Inherent in the concept of "personality disorder" is the idea that the problem is not episodic, as it is in, for instance Snit Disorder, but is constantly present since early adulthood. Once again, the vulnerability to all emotional conditions springs from extraordinary emotional sensitivity and reactivity. However, in Borderline Personality Disorder, the predominant, baseline reaction is not anxiety but anger, and, as mentioned above, anger is an emotion which does not look inwards, but only outwards towards the person who is both source and target of it.

Picture yourself in an intimate relationship in which your overly sensitive "buttons" are being pushed all the time and instead of the baseline reaction being anxiety, it is anger. Anger then becomes a constant, underlying tone in your attitude towards your partner. You are the party who feels chronically abused by constant rejection, and your resentment fuels a long-term campaign to catalogue and vehemently respond to "infractions" when they occur. The expressions of this chronically angry mood usually are not abusive because the intent is not primarily to relieve frustration by projecting hurt, but rather to indoctrinate and convince the partner that his or her behavior is abusive. The Borderline Personality rails against the partner in order to forcefully convince him or her that it is the patient who is being victimized.

The inside of these patients are filled with self-justified resentment for long lists of slights, abandonment and isolation. Fuelled by self-fulfilling rejection, this tragic person is driven to extract from those around him or her behaviors that are loving and affectionate. The penalties for not receiving the pursued responses (which are, in fact, truly needed by the patient) are angry tirades always leaving doubts in these patients about whether the gestures thus extracted are truly meaningful or whether they are they merely fabrications produced to pacify the rage and keep the peace. If I had a poetic bent, I would write an ode to this often ostracized group. These are the "horrible" husbands and wives who have been left behind with good riddance and rejoicing. They are often denied that aspect of life that is most fulfilling: the abiding comfort of a close and intimate relationship.

TREATMENT OF
BORDERLINE PERSONALITY DISORDER

To repeat the vital point, whereas the discomfort caused by the emotions of fear and anxiety is focused within the sufferer, the emotion of anger is focused outside, in this case toward the people who are "causing" rejection. The treatment of Snit

Disorder is facilitated by the fact that it is episodic so that, when the patient is "in the soup," he or she can strive to hold onto the realization that his or her thinking is distorted and the sufferer can "hold his or her breath" until it is over. Even when within a snit, the fear of abandonment predominates. In Borderline Disorder, the anger in response to perceived incidents of rejection by the partner may periodically erupt, but, at all times, it persists as a sort of self-protective "undercoating" for as long as the patient is in an intimate relationship. While the Snit sufferer erupts because the "bone" has been grabbed out of his mouth, the Borderline sufferer simmers endlessly because she feels that she has never gotten the love and affection she needed in the first place.

In order to empathize with the person with Borderline Disorder, one must think of someone for whom one has developed a strong dislike for whatever reason. Just as you would reject the notion that you need therapy to understand why you dislike this person and might conclude that it is he or she who needs help, the person with Borderline Disorder rejects therapy, because the patient is convinced that it is the other person who is the source of the problem.

What is a psychiatrist to do when the "patient" says that it is the partner who is causing all the problems? Conjoint marital (partner) therapy with these patients is usually doomed because there are very few therapists tactful enough (including myself) to get around the trap of being perceived as taking the "wrong" side of the argument. Sooner or later, the therapist is invalidated by the Borderline Personality for the equivalent of settling a dispute between a Republican and a Democrat by declaring one of them sick. These are patients who, if they have the resources and are willing to get help, can benefit from long term, Insight Oriented Psychotherapy with a thoughtful, even-tempered therapist. The Borderline Condition is caused by a constitutionally aggressive temperament causing vulnerability in the formation of healthy attachments in childhood. The therapy relationship itself becomes a laboratory in which the anger can be desensitized and "worked through" to an internal dynamic balance with the underlying fear and anxiety over issues of abandonment. Newer group therapy formats in which the control and management of manipulative anger becomes part of a group effort guided by a therapist makes eminent sense to me as a rational and accessible approach to learning to manage the problem. The bottom line in any therapy is that the patient has to understand and accept that he or she has a problem before it can be effectively treated.

As tough as therapy is with these patients, medication definitely takes second fiddle. Antidepressants can help the patient actively in therapy, and low dose antipsychotic medication can be helpful in an emotional crisis. However, my experience is that the hyper-emotionality generated by marital disputes is not very treatable with medicines. The sheer power in the dynamic of two people emotionally "upping the ante" to a screeching pitch simply "ploughs" right through the buffering effects of medication.

Consideration over time is usually given as to whether the symptoms represent a subtle form Bipolar Disorder because that condition is effectively treated by medication (See Chapter 9). The key issue in this differential diagnosis is whether the outbursts of emotion cycle in and out, with extended periods of time entirely free of problems. I personally do not believe, as some do, that low intensity forms of Bipolar Disorder actually cause true Borderline symptoms as opposed to occasional co-existence.

If I see a young person who manifests this angry hyper-sensitivity in close relationships, as well as recommending psy-chotherapy, I warn the patient that marriage is going to be tough. Those with Borderline Personality Disorder should place at the center of their lives a strong career from which they can draw emotional sustenance with dependability. In addition, putting extra effort into the maintenance of a circle of close friends is helpful lest the elevated emotional needs with which these patients (clients?) are burdened are placed solely upon a single relationship in marriage. Skill in treating this condition is rare and special note should be taken when patients report positive experiences with therapy. Advice should be dispensed to trusted friends who should wait for a receptive moment, when the patient reaches out for help, to then redeem this trust with strong advice to seek competent psychotherapeutic help.

I have attempted to counsel the partners of patients afflicted with Borderline Personality Disorder, but only if they convince me that they truly love their afflicted partners. And, in a dramatic manifestation of how mate selection (perhaps for the benefit of offspring?) delicately and mysteriously balances one temperament with that of another, love them they do. I have attempted to educate these confused individuals about their spouse's condition. I have cautioned them about the so-called "Stockholm syndrome" in which people tend to become "brainwashed" by the uncompromising views of those who hold them hostage. In other words, negative views about the spouse, vigorously expressed over long periods of time (the long memory for misdeeds) tend to sink into their own belief-system about themselves.

I counsel not to get caught up in every single fight, but, rather, to "pick your battles" and stand your ground on important issues. Such issues might be the maintenance of relationships with the partner's own friends and family, which are often seen as a threat by the patient. Timing is everything in discussing these issues. Choose a calm, upbeat moment as opposed to adding fuel to an argument. Most of all, I remind these partners that the source of their spouses' rage is their desperate attachment to them, producing an intolerable state of dependency. Such sufferers are like divers in the sea of life and their spouses the only source of oxygen. Perhaps you alone possess the strength to have been entrusted with the care of someone so fragile on the inside. Perhaps this quaking core, in order to survive at all, must be protected within a shell of rage.

Chapter 6

OBSESSIVE COMPULSIVE DISORDER (OCD)

In Chapter 4, depression is discussed as the brain's shutdown response to the feedback reverberation of two forms of anxiety in the same way fever is a response to an infection. The body has another response to infection, which is to encapsulate it into an abscess in order to isolate it from the rest of the body. OCD can be seen as a similar attempt by the mind to encapsulate anxiety in order to isolate it. However that solution backfires and becomes a deeply entrenched "pocket" of intense feedback reverberation. Generalized anxiety which approaches panic in a young person might attach itself to a fear of infection. Now, theoretically the anxiety can be overcome by avoiding infection, for example by washing his or her hands frequently the patient has finally found a small refuge. However, although the patient's hands are cleaned during the washing process, as soon as the patient touches the knob that others have touched to turn off the water, the anxiety returns. Now the anxiety is intensely focused on the repetition of the hand washing, which further intensifies the anxiety in a feedback reverberation that is the emblem of all mental illness. The patient's generalized anxiety has now been transformed into consumption by a secret behavior. He or she now may wear gloves, not for protection from germs, but to hide their chapped and bleeding hands which have become the object of intense shame.

Anxiety normally serves a problem avoidance function, which scans the future for those paths too risky to traverse. Under most circumstances, anxiety about future problems abates in response to diligent consideration and prudent preparations for them. One prepares to go to bed and makes sure the doors are locked and the stove jets are off. As you walk up stairs, you think to yourself, "Did I turn off those gas jets? I was preoccupied when I did it and do not specifically remember doing it." So you go down and check them again and say to yourself as you check them, "I am now turning off this gas jet." You then go upstairs to deal with your insomnia. This behavior qualifies you to be on my "team" on the anxious side of the population bell curve, but does not "make the cut" for you to be diagnosed with OCD.

When someone with OCD checks those gas jets, it is the fire of his or her anxiety which is the issue. Just like washing the hands, the moment of checking brings relief, but the anxiety of walking away overwhelms any certainty of having just checked it. Who knows, the tight little loop of feedback reverberation involved in this kind of compulsive behavior may actually impair the registration of memories of the checking behavior in the brain. In order to qualify as having OCD, a person has to spend hours involved in these behaviors every day. Checking, straightening, hoarding, the list is large. Any behavior designed to reduce anxiety that as been "short circuited" into extremely excessive repetition qualifies as OCD.

Two Components of OCD

Obsessive Compulsive Disorder has two components. The term, compulsive, refers to outward behavior such as hand washing. The term, obsessive, refers to inner "behavior" in the realm of thought. For example, worrying is a common word for obsessing. Beyond a clinically defined threshold of intensity, worrying can form the underpinning of a chronic anxiety problem that rises to the level of an illness, which, accordingly can underlie chronic depression (see section on Chronicity at the end of Chapter 4). But true OCD differs from the example of worry in its fragmentary nature. I have often compared it to a "broken record[11]," a metaphor which may be incomprehensible to the younger generation. In fact, I have noted a similar phenomenon with compact discs in which a fragment of music suddenly repeats itself over and over again. If you have experienced the mental disruption this causes in listening to music, perhaps you can imagine what it would feel like if that happened with a little piece of a thought brimming with anxiety.

The psychological phenomenon of obsession is the same as with compulsions. A young person may become anxious about his or her sexual identity. The thought, "Maybe I'm gay" becomes the equivalent of checking the gas jets on the stove, except that it is in the person's head "24/7." This person receives a modicum of relief by "monitoring" his or her "gayness," but the anxiety of leaving it "unmonitored" drives its constant repetition. Common obsessions involve anxiety over unacceptable feelings of anger or sexuality that are encapsulated into "worst case" fragments, such as, "I might strangle someone"

---

[11] Referring to the old vinyl records as opposed to modern compact disks (which are probably on the verge of extinction themselves).

or "Maybe I am a whore" being mentally repeated over and over again. The problem is that, once these obsessional "short circuits" are established, they most often tear themselves away from and far outlast the meaning of the fears that initiated them in the first place, to become intransigent, self sustaining "psychiatric abscesses."

TREATMENT OF OCD

It is of utmost importance to read the section in Chapter 3 on Behavior Therapy before proceeding. I believe that an experienced practitioner in Behavior Therapy should take the lead in the treatment of OCD initially with the secondary support of a primary care physician or psychiatrist. Often Cognitive Therapy is lumped with behavior therapy with the catchall phrase, CBT, standing for Cognitive Behavioral Therapy, but I have found that real "nuts and bolts" Behavior Therapy as described in Chapter 3 is hard to find these days. In OCD, the cognitive errors represented by the exaggeration of the actual danger, of germs for example, are fairly straightforward; the hard part is motivating and gradually pushing the patient into creatively individualized exposure and response prevention exercises. Also, when dealing with obsessions, in which everything is truly going on inside the patient's mind, it becomes difficult to define the fear that the obsession is covering up.

Behaviorists believe in the Law of Desensitization and that the compulsive or obsessive behavior has to be wrestled away gradually so that the patient can slowly be desensitized to the resulting anxiety. It is a little bit like an addict going through withdrawal. The goal of treatment is to attempt to get patients to try to gradually expose themselves to the anxiety produced when the behavior is blocked. In the language of Behaviorism, the treatment is "exposure" by means of "response prevention." The most classical and straightforward of these treatments is for a germ phobia in which the fear of germs is perpetuated by the excessive hand washing. The therapeutic instructions, to be done in graduated steps, are to take a handkerchief and to systematically touch all the symbolically "dirty" objects such as door knobs, handles, tires, etc. (usually things that, themselves, touch a lot of other things or people), and then carry the handkerchief around in a pocket, touching it frequently, while limiting hand washing progressively. Sounds odd, but it works and that is the only thing that matters.

An illustration of the effective treatment of OCD in a situation closer to common experience is afforded by advice that I have given patients who are fixated on some out-of-control problem in their life. For example someone suddenly finds himself thrust into being a defendant in a law suit. He can't get it out of his mind, waking up in the middle of the night thinking about it all the time. (This condition would not be diagnosed as OCD because lacks the characteristic fragmentary nature.) The cognitive portion of the treatment is to get patient to agree that obsessing about the problem all the time is not productive in any way: no breakthroughs have resulted in how to deal with the situation producing the anxiety. I instruct them to cordon off a limited period of time once a day, preferably in the morning when the mind is fresh, to think through the problem thoroughly. I suggest to them that the function of obsessing about the problem is to "protect" them from the even greater anxiety of not thinking about it. I explain that maintaining mental "contact" with the problem is similar to a dog watching a squirrel: the fear is that, if one takes one's mind's "eye" off of it, the problem might sneak up behind you and "get you" while you're "asleep at the switch," or in the case of the dog, the squirrel will escape. I never fail to add that the tendency to be anxious and to think carefully about life's possible pitfalls is a personality trait that has served the patient well, but, in this particular situation, it has gotten "out of kilter."[12] I have often given these patients the curious advice to attempt to tolerate the anxiety (exposure) of not thinking about the problem (response prevention) except during the predetermined times.

MEDICATION TREATMENT OF OCD

Unfortunately a significant portion of severe OCD conditions are not tractable to treatment by behavioral methods. These conditions are too entrenched or simply do not lend themselves to desensitization methods. Like all anxiety based illnesses, OCD is helped by the SSRI antidepressants. Prozac (available as fluoxetine) is the most commonly prescribed, but all are helpful. There are three commonly accepted differences in the treatment of particularly severe manifestations of OCD, as opposed to other anxiety and depression conditions. The first is that, usually, the dose needs to be generally higher, as much as three times higher than for other conditions, which is one of the reasons Prozac (available as fluoxetine) is preferred; psychiatrists are generally more comfortable with high doses of fluoxetine because it has been around longer. Secondly, the time

---

[12] I could have said, "out of whack," which evokes commonly accepted verbal slurs on the mentally ill, such as "whack job" or "whacko." I assume there is an equivalent word to "crazy" in every language, delivered replete with smirk and the universal finger pointed towards the head, circling about the ear. Is it possible that, at some distant time, such an ingrained epithet could be banned like racial slurs?

until the patient sees a response is longer: several months instead of several weeks. One needs a higher dose and longer time on an antibiotic to get at an encapsulated abscess, and the same is true of treating its psychiatric equivalent, OCD, with antidepressants.

The tricyclic antidepressant, Anafranil (available as clomipramine), which predominantly effects serotonin, is thought by some to be a more potent anti-OCD medication than the SSRI antidepressants, but with the side effects of dry mouth, constipation, and dizziness upon standing up quickly, possibly causing a risk of falling in the elderly. There are other adjunctive medications, including all classes of tranquillizing medications, and others, which have been used with some success in severe, treatment-resistant cases.

For most mental illnesses successfully treated by medications, the expectation is a full therapeutic remission. The third difference is that in the case of severe OCD, the expectation is for, perhaps a 50% improvement, which most of these terribly suffering patients are happy to accept. Again, in most cases, vigorous concurrent Behavior Therapy can significantly improve the outcome of treatment. After the illness is under control, Insight Oriented Therapy can be helpful to consolidate gains and as a prophylaxis against recurrence.

Chapter 7

Post-Traumatic Stress Disorder (PTSD)

P ost-Traumatic Stress Disorder is an anxiety/panic condition characterized by some variety of re-experiencing or flashback of a traumatic event and the phobic avoidance of circumstances that remind the patient of it. PTSD is like OCD (see Chapter 6 above) "on steroids." Whereas, in OCD, anxiety is reduced to an "abscess" of repetitive behavior, in PTSD, the anxious memory of a traumatic event thrusts itself into the patient's life and expands outwards. Repetitive traumatic memories, such as the "impact feeling" of a car accident, ravenously barges into feedback reverberation with any and all present experiences which can be remotely associated with the trauma.

Controversy has surrounded the designation of the level of severity of trauma that qualifies for the diagnosis of PTSD. This is driven mainly by the attempt to limit legal benefits to those who have suffered varieties of trauma. The role of predisposition is made more obvious in PTSD in that only a minority of people will develop symptoms in response to a given traumatic event, but this is no different than the relationship between predispositions to any other mental illness and the various stresses that precipitate them. Symptoms are symptoms and they need to be treated regardless of the objective magnitude of the precipitating stress.

I have usually felt that the sudden appearance of panic and phobias has a better prognosis (with treatment) if it can be attributable to an identifiable single trauma which is unlikely to be repeated in that the symptoms will predictably fade after a year or two. Expanding symptoms into disruption of the patient's relationships by hysteria (see section on hysteria in Chapter 4) bespeak of the destabilization by the trauma of pre-existing relational vulnerabilities which could be addressed in Insight Oriented Therapy. In such cases, it is well, with some regularity, to indoctrinate the patient's partner in the art and discipline of granting the rights and privileges of patienthood until the symptoms lift.

I myself, as a young psychiatrist, was attacked in a prison by an inmate. The prisoner beckoned me over to his cell, whereupon he cut my cheek clear through with a razor blade; I then looked him in the eye as he attempted to cut my throat, causing a superficial laceration which, had it been deeper, would have severed my jugular vein. I continued working at the prison, because I was determined in my personal mission to examine motivations for criminal behavior. Nonetheless, clanking through those holding cells each day filled me with dread. I continually had to deal with the remembered experience of being attacked, which extended to an attack on my young family. My response was to acquire a second German Shepherd and to construct an impenetrable barbed wire fence around my property. Then, after 18 months of dreadful fear, it went away. I am, therefore very sympathetic to all varieties of odd behavior that these patients tailor to protect themselves from the persistent, anxious haunting by their memories.

Preceded by the terms, "shell shock" and "battle fatigue," awareness of PTSD originated from the extreme, prolonged trauma of war. As opposed to isolated incidents, the length of exposure in spousal (see "Snit Disorder" in Chapter 5) and child abuse broadens and deepens the resulting PTSD pathology. Symptoms that arise from long periods of trauma can last for many years and are best treated by both a therapist and a psychiatrist (usually in a secondary, consulting role) who have made a specialty of PTSD and have had wide experience and specific training. Group therapies are useful for many, but not all. The art of therapy is to begin with calming, supportive techniques that buffer the patient from the traumatic memories. The self relaxation treatments described in Chapter 4 can be a reliable adjunctive treatment. This is followed by a consensual decision about when to commence desensitization by endless repetitions of each and every detail of the trauma in the safety of a quiet office with a trusted therapist. Gradual desensitization from the anxiety elicited by circumstances that are associated with the trauma can also be part of therapy.

Medication treatment is administered in response to the broad array of symptoms that can vary during the course of the illness, sometimes in complex cases ending up with multiple medications from different classes. All the medications used in these cases are described in the Guidebook and can be referenced in the index. Addiction commonly complicates treatment. Chronic, severe PTSD can be among the most intransigent of mental illnesses.

Chapter 8

ADDICTION, COMPULSION AND IMPULSE CONTROL

W hen I gave lectures to medical students early in the morning, I felt that I had to get their attention somehow. For one of the lectures, I would start with a teasing, "shaggy dog" story. "Today you are going to hear certainly the most important thing you will learn on your psychiatry rotation, and it could be one of the most important things you learn in medical school; period." In my attempt to arouse their attention, I would continue to ramble: "If you really learned what I am going to tell you in just a few minutes and were able to effectively put it into practice, you could almost hang up a shingle and practice psychiatry with just that one piece of information, and, I absolutely guarantee that it will be of substantial use regardless of what specialty you enter." By this time I could usually detect that a stirring of curiosity had penetrated the early morning student torpor.

I proceeded to explain to these medical students that Psychiatry is, at least at this point in time, a rather fuzzy field, and there is really only one hard and fast rule. That rule is: if a psychiatric patient presents with symptoms that could be physical in origin, that possibility must be checked out first. If a person has anxiety and chest pain, a doctor never assumes the chest pain is caused by the anxiety, he or she first orders an electrocardiogram to make sure the patient is not actually having a heart attack. A vitally important corollary of this rule concerns alcohol. If a patient presents with any of the full gamut of psychiatric symptoms from marital squabbling to hearing voices from Mars, and everything in between, and, in the course of conducting the interview, "tucked away in the corner" is significant alcohol consumption, the rule is not that all psychiatric symptoms will get better if the patient stops drinking. The rule is that the psychiatric symptoms will not improve if the patient does not stop drinking. It is a priority rule. If a patient displays an array of confusing symptoms plus excessive drinking, the initial treatment by the doctor must include stopping the drinking, although there are numbers of severe psychiatric conditions that should be treated simultaneously with the cessation of alcohol. The main point is that most psychiatric treatments, including psychotherapy, will not work if there is significant, ongoing drinking. It is important that patients understand this rule early in the healing process, because, my experience has been that, once addiction is pushed aside by other problems and their treatments, I somehow gradually lost my doctorly authority to effectively address it. I have broken this rule many times even as I pontificated to those medical students almost invariably to the detriment of my patients.

ALCOHOLISM

The predilection for alcohol has been with humans since an astute collection of our far distant ancestors, having eaten fermenting fruit picked up from the ground in autumn, put "2 and 2 together." Just exactly what is excessive drinking? Here, we are talking about the psychiatric effects of alcohol, as opposed to the myriad adverse physical effects, most famously on the liver. The rule of thumb is that one drink a day is fine, two a day is moderate and three or more is excessive. It seems that many can "get away" with three drinks a day, but not many past the age of 50. On the other hand, one glass of red wine is purported to be therapeutic. It must be remembered that just the act of drinking is not necessarily a medical or psychiatric problem. Many people get upset with drinking because they have been traumatized by such problems in their family of origin. In order to motivate someone to stop drinking, concrete, adverse physical or, in this case, psychiatric consequences must be pointed out with clarity. Sometimes there will be obvious signs, such as "blackouts," or gross personality changes while drinking. For example, a reserved person suddenly starts talking a "mile a minute" with inappropriate remarks, or an ordinarily nice person becomes mean, withdrawn or sullen. But most often, the problems are far more subtle.

In the days before penicillin, Syphilis was known as the "great pretender" because it could produce symptoms that could mimic many other illnesses, thereby throwing off even the most astute diagnostician. Alcoholism is the "great pretender" in psychiatry. Years of excessive drinking can insinuate itself throughout the patient's personality structure, subtly exaggerating pre-existing weak points in ways that seem to be a natural extension of the personality. Most of these symptoms occur not while the patient is intoxicated, but during the daily withdrawal phase, and include irritability, anxiety and increased stress. These symptoms are often mistaken as normal reactions to the "slings and arrows of outrageous fortune," which "deserve" drinks again at night. What the patient does not understand is that the drinks at night are producing the subtle mood problem during the day, for which the drinks in the evening are the perfect cure. The cure then produces the same symptoms the following day, etc. The patient does not realize that the problems, which are relieved by the drinks tonight are caused by the drinks last night.

In terms of compromising function, family relationships are more sensitive and work is more resistant to alcohol addiction. All the issues make sense, and one can talk about them until blue in the face, but if the drinking does not stop, the symptoms and family dysfunction do not stop. It is not that these problems always go away immediately when the drinking stops (although this does happen), but stopping the alcohol allows the other treatments to work. Stopping drinking is the "cover charge" of psychiatric treatment. I will sometime "bargain" with a patient to see if I can get them to stop drinking for, say 6 weeks, and then promise to "renegotiate." Often six weeks off alcohol is enough time to illustrate specific benefits to the patient and the family such that it provides a "foot in the door." If I am convinced of the problem, I will offer patients my patented "money back guarantee." I promise that my fee will be repaid in full, "cash on the barrel-head" if, having stopped drinking for a year, their lives have not steadily improved according to any standards they wish to choose. If this sounds a little too cute, its only purpose is to express my certainty about the issue.

It is particularly important for friends and family to understand that it is most often exceedingly difficult to stop drinking and it has nothing to do with weakness of personality. I have witnessed people with international reputations for strength of character simply be unable to stop drinking. As we go along in life, we feel reasonably certain that, although we may vacillate back and forth a little, our motivations basically spring from a single source. People who are trapped in alcoholism have developed a second source of motivation in their brain that has a "one track" mind: it wants the patient to drink. When the patient is in my office, listening to my spiel about stopping drinking, that little second source of motivation goes into "hiding" for a while, but it is just waiting to jump out and "suggest" to the patient: "Hey, wouldn't this be the perfect time for just one drink?" The "control room" is then promptly handed over, lock, stock and barrel until the bedraggled patient looks in the mirror the next morning and says, "Today is going to be a different day." Many patients with alcoholism seem to keep alive the fiction that they could stop any time they want but simply do not choose to do so.

DETOXIFICATION

We all must be reminded that Delirium Tremens (DT's) is a serious, occasionally life-threatening condition which should be considered when anyone suddenly stops drinking. The older the patient and the larger the quantity of consumption, the higher should be the concern. The key question is whether or not the person has ever had physical difficulties (sweating or shaking) when they have stopped in the past, because the intensity of DT's usually slowly increases in response to episodes of stopping drinking over the years. Nevertheless, if a patient has a history of significant alcohol intake, it is well that the cessation of drinking be supervised by a medical doctor with the administration of benzodiazepine tranquilizers for at least several days. If the patient has had DT's in the past, admission to a hospital for several days might be warranted. It can be a nightmare for the alcoholic patient to "get behind the curve" of DT's having been admitted for surgery 3 or 4 days earlier, to become delirious with an agitation of such profound proportions that it is only able to be calmed by prolonged administration of huge doses of tranquilizing drugs.

TREATMENT OF ALCOHOLISM

The bottom line in the treatment of a drinking problem is to get the patient simply not to drink. I feel that addiction problems in general, along with eating disorders and Post-Traumatic Stress Disorder, should be treated by specialists in these respective areas. It is particularly important with alcoholism, because of the "priority rule" I mentioned above. Speaking from experience, there is a great tendency for a general psychiatrist or therapist to succumb to the patient's unconscious tendency to draw the therapeutic interchange away from the subject of drinking in favor of much more interesting life events. If a patient walks into an addiction specialist's office, there is really only one item on table, and the patient cannot get around it. Alcoholism is a disease which "sits on your shoulder and tells you that you don't have it." Any significant improvement in this condition must be preceded by the patient's acknowledgement that drinking is, indeed, a problem that the patient can not control alone, which is the first "step" of Alcoholics Anonymous (AA).

It has been said that AA is the most positive social movement to come out of the 20th century. It is a grassroots, folk movement with a down to earth spiritual dimension. AA is a people's movement, with evolving, disseminated wisdom into which no "experts" are allowed to wander, and I intend to respect those boundaries. From the outside, I have observed magical transformations rendered through immersion into this culture too numerous to recall. I have appreciated the humor in the numerous catch phrases, my favorite being, "There is nothing so bad that a drink can't make it worse." When patients with alcohol problems are apprehensive about the "brain washing" aspect of AA, I have occasionally responded, "Perhaps that is precisely what your brain needs." Finally, it has been fashionable in some circles to object to anything which smacks of God, even in the generic "higher power" AA form. It has seemed to me that the spiritual dimension is a central aspect of the program, and I have even advised doubters to "fake it 'til you make it." I have personally witnessed many times AA effectively address the personality "rot" (self centeredness, etc.) that inevitably accompanies addiction.

Some people start going to AA meetings as a guest of an "old timer," but it is much easier to integrate into the program after first attending a supervised inpatient rehabilitation clinic. Traditionally, the gold standard for addiction treatment has been attendance at a 30-day inpatient rehabilitation facility. I believe that it is more effective if the rehabilitation center is a considerable distance from the patient's home, not only because he or she cannot just walk out and go home, but also because it adds to the therapeutic mystique of a "going to the mountain" transformation. Sometimes further "residential" treatment is needed away from home for severe cases. After inpatient care, it is vitally important that there is a seamless transition to an addiction specialist in the patient's locality with attendance at local AA meetings. More than once I have found myself actually hoping that a young person, eaten up with destructive self-involvement, is also afflicted with addiction, because that could then "buy" him or her a ticket of admission to the healing world of AA.

There are addiction therapists who are specialists in conducting "interventions" in which many family members and trusted friends are organized to descend on the unsuspecting patient and to give well thought out, heartfelt appeals for immediate transfer to a residential rehabilitation program. I have seen this work many times, but I have also seen it fail with negative consequences. Three caveats should be kept in mind when contemplating intervention. First there must be strong, concrete evidence that drinking is having disastrous consequences in the patient's life. Second, the marital relationship must be basically strong; the spouse should not be "headed out the door." Third, care should be taken to evaluate whether the patient also has significant other mental illness, and if it is present, the patient should be in a hospital setting in which both problems can be treated simultaneously followed by close post-hospital care for both problems.

The AA program is so convinced that the family is central to the recovery of the alcoholic that there is a sister organization called Al-Anon expressly for family members. Their basic advice, mainly to spouses, is to "detach" from the whole issue of the drinking problem and to focus on functioning in their own lives. Conversely, as the recovering alcoholic starts taking back more responsibility in the family after many years of "absence," spousal adjustments often need to be discussed. Both AA and Al-Anon are focused on problems resulting from excessive mutual dependence, or "co-dependency," and stress taking back responsibility for one's own life.

TREATMENT OF ALCOHOLISM WITH MEDICINES

Medications are a decided side-show in the treatment of alcoholism. Antabuse (available as disulferam) is a very controversial drug which has been used in the treatment of alcoholism for a half a century. It works by blocking the metabolism of alcohol at the point that a very toxic chemical is produced which causes flushing, nausea, and in some instances, cardiovascular collapse and even death. The idea behind this medication is that taking this pill extends early morning resolve not to drink into a whole-day reality (actually, the effect can last up to 3 days) that if you do drink, you will get very sick. Antabuse, particularly at doses over 250mg, can occasionally cause neuropathy in the legs and liver problems. Some patients are so afflicted by alcoholism that they end up drinking with full knowledge that they will get sick. Nevertheless, many patients who are properly motivated, find that taking an Antabuse tablet, even episodically, when they think that they are going to be particularly tempted to drink, is very helpful in taking the issue off the table for several days. Recently, drugs have been introduced that have the effect of lowering alcohol cravings, and they have shown promise in selected patients. At this point, the drug treatment of addiction should be administered by a specialist.

As previously discussed, the patient might also suffer from another mental illness in addition to alcoholism. This so-called "dual diagnosis" might not become apparent until weeks or even months after the mind has adjusted to the absence of alcohol. Significant anxiety and depression can be treated with antidepressants, but an attempt is made to avoid benzodiazepine tranquillizers because they are addictive. Again, the advice I have given to those medical students I feel bears repeating: OTHER PSYCHIATRIC PROBLEMS WILL NOT BE TREATED EFFECTIVELY UNLESS A CO-EXISTING ADDICTION PROBLEM IS RESOLVED FIRST.

OTHER ADDICTIONS

As I have just said, addiction should be treated by an addiction specialist. To me, the "amotivational" syndrome is the problem with marijuana. My image of the chronic pot smoker is a young person, having slid through college, is living in his or her parent's basement, and is just not getting their life off the ground. Lighting up a joint every day enables the marijuana addict to transform his existential anxiety about his life not going anywhere into portentous feelings about himself (while listening to music). Sometimes I have pointed out that the pot smoker "drains" positive feelings that are normally spread throughout the day and concentrates them into a couple of hours at night. My experience is that this wears thin after numbers of years and falls away of its own weight.

Heroin, and narcotics in general, are the "Queen of the addictions." The brain secretes its own narcotic endorphins, which play an integral role in normal function, and, as anyone who has been in extreme pain can attest, narcotics can arrive as on the "wings of angels." As in all addictions, the patient is trapped by the anticipation of dreaded withdrawal effects, which, although not life threatening, are excruciatingly painful. Questions of chronic maintenance on methadone or the newer synthetic combination drugs are complex and should be made on an individual basis by a specialist in addiction. Whereas some people can "get by" in life while addicted to alcohol, pot, or heroin, no one gets away with daily cocaine or methamphetamine abuse. I mentioned that addictions create a separate motivational center in the addicted brain which stealthily and single-mindedly plots to ingest the substance regularly. Cocaine and methamphetamine quickly transform its hapless victims into disgusting, selfish, and sometimes dangerous pigs. In general, the shorter the time between the administration of a substance, and the perception of its effect, the more addictive it is. One feels the effect of alcohol minutes after a drink, but with cigarettes, it is seconds. This "quick hit" effect makes tobacco extremely addictive. Nicotine is a stimulant but does not have major psychiatric effects. The main problem is that smoking can kill you. For addiction to nicotine, group programs that "throw the psychological book at you" from every conceivable angle are most effective. Adjunctive drug therapy that suppresses cravings can be helpful, but usually not without organized support.

EATING DISORDERS

The premise that eating disorders are similar to addictions is complicated by the fact that simple abstinence is not an option. Patients with Anorexia will tell you that not eating is a "high," and that binge eating leaves those with Bulimia an with an intolerable "heavy" feeling only relieved by vomiting or taking laxatives. Nowhere is interplay between psychological concepts of impulsivity and compulsivity more apparent than in eating disorders which lie on a continuum between the two. Theoretically, an impulsive behavior is driven by pleasure (addiction), and a compulsive one by the avoidance of anxiety. However, the basic biology of eating is extremely complex and poorly understood. Clearly, past a certain threshold, aspects of this biological circuitry of hunger and satiation lock into one another in reverberating circuitry, driving these behaviors at an organic level well below that of the patient's psychology. In other words, the psychology of anxious, compulsive perfectionism can drive a young woman to excessive dieting, but then a pathological process takes over at a biological level. The delusional conviction of an emaciated, 80 pound girl with Anorexia that she is fat can be compared to a patient with Melancholic Depression proclaiming that his life is over. Similarly, the binge-purge cycle in Bulimia has deeper, more complex biological roots than mere addictions or compulsions.

TREATMENT OF EATING DISORDERS

Similar to addictions, and Post-Traumatic Stress Disorder, the treatment of eating disorders should be done by a specialist. Also similar to addiction is the patient's denial that there is a problem and resistance to seeking treatment. As always, timing is important. While friends and family wait for an appropriate moment to insist that the patient seek treatment, considerable research must be done concerning treatment options partly because they seem to be constantly in a state of flux. Severe

Anorexia or Bulimia can be life-threatening and hospitalization is sometimes necessary.

Again similar to the treatment of addiction, the central focus of the treatment, starting right at the beginning, has to be directed at the disordered behavior itself. In-patient settings are very structured and centered on gaining weight for Anorexia and blocking purging behavior in Bulimia. The transition home is often difficult and should be immediately followed up with regular visits to a local therapist. A good eating disorder therapist must be able to patiently but relentlessly confront the disordered behavior while at the same time compassionately engaging and supporting the patient. A good doctor is tough on the illness and kind to the patient, but that is particularly difficult to do with eating disordered patients. Effective therapy for eating disorders proceeds slowly with gradual progress. Effective psychotherapy can be compared to orthodontics: if you push on a tooth with all your might for a short time, it does not move, but if you apply slow, steady pressure over a long period of time, it does. Involvement by a nutritionist who has experience with eating disordered patients is often useful. Prozac (available as fluoxetine) and other SSRI antidepressants are an accepted adjunctive treatment, but seem to be most effective in stabilizing gains after the worst part of the behavior has been controlled by effective psychotherapy.

Needless to say eating disorders can be a time of crises for the family and friends of the patient. For friends, simple loyalty is what is needed. For family, the goal is progressive disengagement from the illness, as the patient engages in treatment, but that is easier said than done. For parents living with a young woman with an eating disorder, the inevitable recruitment into the role as "food police" while maintaining that of the sympathetic parent of a sick child can be like riding a bucking bronco. Family therapy can be helpful for this harrowing experience, if only to provide an occasional hour to "come up for air" in an atmosphere of decreased emotional "static."

SEXUAL DISORDERS

Varieties of sexual disorders also lie on a spectrum between impulsive behavior driven by pleasure (addiction) and compulsive behavior driven by the avoidance of anxiety. Also somewhat similar to eating disorders for women, the biology of male sexuality is somehow more intensively looped back in on itself in a reverberated circuit of increasing need for repetition of sexual stimulation. Internet pornography has emerged to feed sexual addictive compulsions, which, it should be pointed out, is much safer than most other kinds of sexual pathology. I cannot suppress the unflattering image of the laboratory rodent in the experimental cage furiously pushing on the little bar that stimulates the electrode in the pleasure center of its brain. Nowhere does the "law" of first controlling pertain more. This is definitely a field for skilled specialists who are able to balance the proffering of insight into the anxiety producing the compulsive aspect, with the more active pushing of the patient out of the addictive aspect. As the therapist moves into areas of sex (and aggression), difficulties arise because usually someone else besides the patient is intimately affected by the pathology.

* * *

Whenever someone starts criticizing the pharmaceutical industry, I respond, "How about Viagra?" In the pre-Viagra psychiatric universe hardly a month went by without a tortured revelation of an incidence of Erectile Dysfunction most often induced by anxiety. Then, "poof," an ancient scourge, along with all its remedies like Spanish fly, ground up rhinoceros horns, and years of psychoanalysis, quietly evaporated. The word "impotence" also made a quiet exit. In the "war between the sexes," the significance of Viagra for men easily rivals the advent of birth control for women.

Routine office advice concerning sexual difficulties involves explaining that sometimes a loving, sympathetic relationship is necessary for a good sexual relationship: "Maybe you are just too sensitive for casual sex." For the "he wants it more than she does" problem, pick a compromise frequency and both secretly conspire to make it happen. The doctor sternly adds, "To keep a marriage healthy, you should be having sex on a regular basis." Then after an appropriate pause, a gratuitous statistic is appended: "The national average is once a week." Serious sexual dysfunction is best dealt with by a trained specialist with both partners involved.

Chapter 9

BIPOLAR DISORDER

Social animals, such as dogs and primates definitely suffer from Atypical Depression, and may even experience a rudimentary form of Melancholic Depression (the poor rat in the jar of water), but only humans are afflicted by mania and Schizophrenia. In order for the diagnosis of Bipolar Disorder to be made, it is necessary to reliably diagnose a manic state in a patient. "Unipolar" mania is rarely seen, but typically, patients who have manic episodes, also have depression, hence the term Bipolar. The participation of a representative from the patient's family and friends is nowhere more important than in the diagnosis and treatment of Bipolar Disorder because, similar to alcohol or drug addiction, mania is often not identified by the patient as problematic at all.

Classical, full blown mania is one of the most dramatic presentations in all of medicine and can be a family's worst nightmare come true. It can erupt quite suddenly for no apparent reason or build up over a period of weeks. Think of the sweepstakes man knocking on your door one night and, with cameras popping, he hands you a check for a hundred million dollars. Suddenly, you are on a high. You call up all your friends and can not stop talking through the night. Your plans expand from buying a few new cars and houses, and then, perhaps giving money to a politician, but, then again, why give it to him when I, myself, could run for office and pursue world peace more directly? In its pure form, like addictions, mania is fed by the feedback reverberation of euphoric pleasure, in this condition, that of social approbation. The mania is emotionally driven by feelings that can be likened to daily being honored by lifetime achievement awards, to being promoted to the highest level in your company, to buying only the best with witty sexuality exuding from every pore. It sometimes is impossible not to be drawn in to the hilarity of such a revved up caricature of the inner peacock inside us all.

But very quickly, this entertaining picture reveals the darkness of a devastating sickness. The patient is not sleeping; his racing thoughts and actions are increasingly fragmented, starting one thing and then repeatedly distracted into others; often the grandiosity hardens into fixed delusion, or, more alarming, irritability can grow into menacing flash rage states that emerge when the patient is "crossed" or interrupted and then metastasize into embattled paranoia. Not uncommonly, these floridly psychotic patients strenuously resist the idea that they are sick and in need of help. Sometimes, the family, friends and doctors are forced into settling for merely keeping in contact with the patient, like a fish too large to reel in. They find themselves hoping for some minor transgression, just enough to justify authorities to take the patient to a hospital instead of jail. A collection of experienced policeman who can exert a gentle "show of force" can be more effective than a team of "shrinks" in effectively transporting a floridly manic patient to an appropriate in-patient treatment setting.

On the other end of the spectrum of mania, it is not uncommon for episodes of "hypo-mania" to be brief and subtle.

Because these periods are often experienced by the patient himself as being "up" and remembered as positive, the physician may need the patient's partner to assist in probing more deeply as to whether the patient's behavior was a bit too expansive; was there an incremental loss of normal judgment with respect to spending habits or sundry behavior which crossed interpersonal boundaries normally observed. Manic mental states are sometimes difficult to diagnose, and friends and family can play a crucial role in the prevention of a misdiagnosis because the stakes are high. If the diagnosis is falsely made, this needlessly obligates the patient to take powerful mood stabilizing medicines, some with serious side effects. If the diagnosis of mania is missed and the patient proceeds to cycle into depression, treatment with antidepressants could make the entire illness worse, perhaps even permanently.

The depression side of Bipolar Disorder is normally much longer lasting than the manic side and far more distressing to the patient. Most commonly, the depression consists mainly of the pure shutdown symptoms of starkly diminished will power. It has seemed to me that the manic state had overwhelmed, but also stimulated the shutdown mechanism such that, after the mania has burned itself out, it continues in a hypertrophied form, dominating the patient's mental state. Even after the patient finally recovers from depression, subsequently ever milder, shorter and subtle recurrences of hypomania can trip a lowered threshold to reawaken another extended bout of depression.

Sometimes patients "hang onto" some of the grandiose notions they cherished when they were high, but the experience is usually remembered with a painful, longing mix, like a whirlwind romance that ended with a jilt. When "drive reversal" (see above) or tons of guilt directed inwards is present, it is possible that the patient suffers from both Melancholic Depression and Bipolar Disorder, which may lead the psychiatrist to weigh the risks of treating the depression more aggressively. Treating depression in a patient with known Bipolar Disorder is one of the most difficult treatments in psychiatry because antidepressants can precipitate a manic state. Advice to family and friends of patients in the depression phase of Bipolar Disorder is to encourage patience and realistic hope that the depression will slowly improve with persistent treatment. Although difficult, the treatment of Bipolar Disorder is, perhaps, psychiatry's greatest success story, as shall be described below.

The fact that antidepressants can precipitate mania is further evidence that functional emotional entities in the mind exist in dynamic balance with each other. The classic Prozac "makeover," which astounded many after it was first introduced, consisted of making people less anxious, less socially inhibited, and more able to be "out there" in their lives. Clearly, social anxiety functions as a restraint on extroverted, manic-tinged tendencies in patients who are pushed into mania by antidepressants. I find it useful to think in terms of the basic directionality of emotion: Like gravity, obsessive anxiety binds its thoughts in repetitive orbits to the patient, tightly holding everything in place. The basic force is pressing inwards. Released from the restraint of anxiety, mania thrusts its patients out within their thoughts and drives them on a joy-ride, leaping with excitement from one idea to the next and then the next. The basic force of mania is branching outwards.

MIXED STATE BIPOLAR DISORDER

Unfortunately, particularly when some patients have been on antidepressants for a while, depression can occasionally devolve into a dual feedback reverberation producing a very painful "mixed state" in which the racing aspect of mania coexists with the anxiety of obsessive thinking. The incidence of these difficult to diagnose and treat mixed states has definitely increased since the wide spread use of SSRI antidepressants, and there is wide suspicion that they are implicated. For this reason, if a patient, who is being treated with antidepressants even without the prior diagnosis of Bipolar Disorder, experiences a shift into racing thoughts and agitation, it is important that this be communicated to or referred to a psychiatrist. It is as if the antidepressant shifted the balance from anxiety regulating mania to a smoldering form of mania dominating, which then re-stimulates anxiety.

TREATMENT OF BIPOLAR DISORDER

As mentioned above, once a manic state has been positively identified by a psychiatrist, from that moment on, treatment with medication is predominately with mood stabilizers. Psychiatry's first "miracle" drug was lithium, widely in use since the 1960's. Lithium, unlike any other psychiatric drug is a simple salt, like you put on food. It is not metabolized by the liver, so it does not interact with other drugs except for diuretics, which can make the level of lithium increase. The best thing about lithium is that only very rarely are there adverse psychiatric reactions to it;[13] it does not make the patient jittery, groggy or anything like that because it a simple salt.

Psychiatrically, lithium has broad stabilizing and even mild antidepressant effects, and adding just a little bit of lithium to an established stabilizing treatment regimen is virtually always a small step in the right direction. The problem with lithium is that its therapeutic blood level is close to its toxic level, so that obtaining blood levels are necessary to adjust it properly. Too much lithium causes tremors and diarrhea. Also, long-term administration can cause thyroid and kidney changes which need to be monitored at least once a year. Many patients have been stable for many years on lithium after tumultuous episodes of mania when they were young. Lithium levels should be checked more frequently in the elderly because decreasing kidney function can slowly increase the lithium level in the system to toxic levels.

After lithium was first identified as an effective treatment for mania, it was demonstrated that some anticonvulsants used for epilepsy also have effective anti-manic effects. Depakote (generic, valproic acid, is rarely used) has been a central mood stabilizing medicine for many years. A collection of side effects, such as weight gain, sedation, occasional liver and kidney problems, hair loss, plus a relatively high level of birth defects if taken during pregnancy make it less than ideal. Also, Depakote does not help the depressive side of the illness. Often the psychiatrist is pushed by the patient's depression grinding on for months, to cautiously add small doses of an antidepressant, beneath the "cover" of, perhaps, several mood stabilizers in order to prevent the "breakthrough" of another

---

[13] Occasionally a patient, often a lawyer, has told me that they feel that lithium takes the "edge" off the sharpness of their thinking.

manic state. Wellbutrin SR (available as bupropion SR) is a popular antidepressant to use in this situation because it is stimulating and has been thought to be less liable to precipitate mania. The use of many medicines simultaneously is the rule in these complex treatments, often spanning many years.

More recently, in an important development, the anticonvulsant, Lamictal (generic: lamotrogine) was approved for the prevention of depression in Bipolar patients. This drug provides for the first time a weapon against the depressive side of the Bipolar condition. Particularly attractive is that most (not all) who take this medication have no side effects and it is "weight neutral."[14] The very important exception is that the drug can occasionally cause a potentially fatal rash (Stevens-Johnson's Syndrome), which, if it goes unnoticed can overwhelm the patient. The risk is approximately 1 in 5,000. However, this drug, like many other drugs, also has approximately a 10% incidence of non-dangerous rashes. This means that, if a patient develops any rash, the drug is immediately stopped and the patient must to be checked out by a dermatologist who has been alerted in advance that the patient may need emergency consultation. The risk of rash can be minimized by extremely slowly increasing the dose such that it may take over a month to achieve a therapeutic level. Most patients who have struggled with bipolarity for years are more than willing to take these kinds of risks and will meticulously follow these instructions. Lamictal has helped many finally stabilize from the disruption of constant mood swings, but, alas, not all.

The other class of medications that has been effective for Bipolar Disorder is the Atypical Antipsychotic medications.

---

[14] Unfortunately, almost all psychiatric medicines cause weight gain, some more than others.

These are medicines originally developed for the treatment of Schizophrenia. They are called "atypical" to contrast them with the older "classical" antipsychotics such as Thorazine (available as chlorpromazine) and Haldol (available as haloperidol). Risperdal (available as risperidone), Zyprexa (generic olanzepine), Seroquel (generic quetiapine), and Geodon (generic: ziprasidone) are valuable tranquillizing and mood stabilizing medications for the short term stabilization of agitation in manic states. Zyprexa, particularly, is an excellent, broad spectrum tranquilizing medication which can be used by the physician for virtually any agitated state to safely, reliably, and appropriately calm the patient down within about an hour.

With prolonged use, these drugs, have been proven effective in stabilizing Bipolar symptoms, but have been shown to cause significant weight gain (particularly Zyprexa and Seroquel), and can precipitate diabetes in predisposed patients. Abilify (generic: aripiprazole) is also in this group. It has a novel dopamine modulating effect, is not sedating, does not have the weight gain problem, and has been approved for use as a mood stabilizer. For a more detailed description of these medications, see Chapter 11. As complex as these bipolar treatments can be, eventually, again with the vital ingredient of dogged persistence, most arrive at a point of stability with combinations of medications and proceed to live their lives with a stable mood for which they are very thankful.

Family support is especially important in the treatment of Bipolar Disorder. Needless to say, having a spouse "swinging from the chandeliers" at one time and moping around most of the rest, is almost as disruptive for the family as it is for the patient. The family needs to inform themselves about the nature of this illness. They need to support the patient in the persistent commitment to medical treatment. They also need to be involved, most specifically, as mentioned, in helping identify the patient's unique pattern of "early warning" symptoms of an impending manic episode, which remain constant over time, such as not sleeping, talking or buying too much, etc. Especially early in the disease process, the patient's family can help the patient into the realization that, in this condition, feeling too good is a bad sign.

It is widely thought that careful regulation of the patient's sleeping habits, including care about the sleep disruption involved in travel, can help prevent a recurrence of mania. Not sleeping works to push the patient into mania. Generally, with some exceptions, over the very long haul, if the mania can be controlled, the depression will eventually go away on its own. This is because, in my judgment, the manic aspect, no matter how minor and brief it may become, triggers an increasingly "hypertrophied" shutdown response which then instantiates itself for long periods as depression. Your house keeps burning down, so you install an elaborate, industrial grade sprinkling system. Now, whenever you light a match, it starts raining and you can't turn the damn thing off. The patient just has to live without "playing with fire" at all, including being very careful with drinking alcohol, which goes together with mania like "love and marriage." All this places a heavy load on a family, but, God bless them, most seem to manage somehow.

Chapter 10

SCHIZOPHRENIA

Schizophrenia[15] is the most difficult to understand of all the mental illnesses because the symptoms of those afflicted seem so removed from any normal experience. Other mental illnesses, such as Panic, depression, Obsessive Compulsive Disorder, or mania, are usually much easier for the ordinary person to relate to, because they have components of normal behavior. In the case of mania for example, the experience of "getting carried away" with oneself, going on a spending spree, or talking too much after a drink or two is well within common experience. Mania and Schizophrenia, which are exclusively human illnesses, can be distinguished by the basic "directionality" of emotion.

"VOICES"

In Mania, all thought is poring outwards in a torrential performance into which the patient disappears. In Schizophrenia, however, it is the patient who is the audience.

---

[15]The word, bedlam, was coined by 16th century London society who would amuse themselves by watching the insane from public balconies in Bethlem Hospital. In 1793, the founder of modern psychiatry, Phillipe Pinel, ordered the chains removed from the insane inside the Paris prisons. If you are ever at Williamsburg Village in Virginia, a visit to the "Pubic House" will give you a graphic view of how the mentally ill were treated in colonial times.

The hallmark of Schizophrenia is the hallucinatory perception of voices. The patient may be the recipient of, or, maybe, just "overhear" a variety of other forms of messages or be privy to distorted circumstances happening all around which are experienced as "directed" at the patient. Characteristically, although these communications are highly meaningful to the patient, they make no sense at all to others. In Schizophrenia, the emotional function that becomes "unglued" involves that of belief. That belief involves emotion is not normally appreciated. We can most clearly see the emotions of belief manifested in religion or politics, but systems of belief motivate individuals in many group activities from patriotic pursuits, professional, or businesslike activities, or even living according to a certain family ethic. The emotional force exerted by group "belief systems" could be compared to the gravitational force the sun, imperceptibly preventing the earth from flying off in space, while at the same time illuminating our entire verbal world of symbols. Perhaps we could say that our belief systems exert their influence upon us more like constellations of stars all relatively fixed in their consistent pulling on us. We have no perception of this emotional mechanism because, when it is functioning, we are its willing instruments. We act according to certain principles because we are as immersed in the emotions of our beliefs as we are within the air we breathe.

In Schizophrenia, the neural mechanisms whereby, minute by minute and second by second, these "group emotions" are transmitted within the individual are "short circuited" and spin off into feedback reverberation. The illness often becomes an enthralling social experience all inside the patient's mind. It competes with normal social contact and often contributes to isolation. Indeed a prominent sign of Schizophrenia is that the patient falls out of accepted social systems. The structures we all take for granted, such as those of political and economic authority or that of social status are fragmented and distorted in those afflicted with this illness.

In talking to each other, we string together thoughts, one following logically after the next. Our belief systems are communicated in the background, constantly, altogether as a whole. Thus, when a patient relates the inner experience of this illness, to the listener it makes no sense. The patient may jump repeatedly from one thing to something completely unrelated, but to the patient these thoughts carry with them the intense feelings of conviction. These internal experiences are driven by the emotion of belief, which has escaped regulation and has been thrown onto a state of feedback reverberation. The common experience most closely resembling Schizophrenia is dreaming during which emotional aspects of our normal lives, which are invisible while we are awake, propel us into a virtual world of nonsensical juxtaposition of events which are, none the less, saturated with the emotional belief that they are real.

The function which becomes distorted and hyperactive in Schizophrenia has to do with thinking rather than talking. Talking is something that we do in order to "display" our thoughts to others. We can also talk to ourselves, but much of thinking is something that happens to us, as if from the outside, in response to our surroundings, jogging memories, which then jog others. An enlightening moment came when I asked a woman, whom I had known for many years in treatment for longstanding Schizophrenia, how she managed to drive a car with constant voices talking to her. Her response was simple: "Don't you think or daydream when you are driving, Dr. Wylie?" Patients with Schizophrenia, when they are not absorbed into a florid, agitated episode, are able to communicate adequately, for the moment, ignoring the "loud thoughts" or compelling beliefs occurring in their mind.

The course of untreated Schizophrenia is marked by sporadic episodes of agitated confusion. Following these episodes, the generic shutdown response can be seen during which the so-called "negative" symptoms of Schizophrenia — the lack of will to do anything and even a dearth of thinking activity itself — may predominate. However, beyond these acute shutdown symptoms, seen in the depressive aspect of many psychiatric conditions, this illness causes a chronic disengagement from the drive for social status and economic pursuit, which consumes so much of ordinary life. As the condition stabilizes into its chronic form, the sometimes subtle "short circuiting" of these social motivations in the patient's thinking process achieves a pathological stability. In response to the mental hyperactivity of continuous feedback reverberation, the resultant shutdown response (often called emotional "flatness") causes a chronic double disability. It is as if the neural traffic which underlies the patient's thinking has blazed shortcuts with overbuilding through several little neighborhoods which then drain the energy from the city as a whole.

Paradoxically, the sudden onset of a wildly psychotic episode in a young person can have a better prognosis for eventual improvement and even complete recovery than the more ominous gradual appearance of social isolation and a slowly developing eccentric inner world that edges toward delusion and paranoia. Family and friends must carefully mix hope with reality when contemplating the future of a young person who has been reliably diagnosed with Schizophrenia over a period of months and years. There is no cure for Schizophrenia. The medications are of inestimable comfort for the harshest "fevers" of this ancient scourge but the underlying condition persists in many. Because Schizophrenia impairs abilities to negotiate the intricate social politics of life, the patient needs protection from it. Common goals are independent living in loosely supervised group housing and sheltered working situations often run by nonprofit organizations supported and enlivened by dedicated family members of afflicted patients.

TREATMENT OF SCHIZOPHRENIA

It is particularly difficult to become comfortable conversing with people who are afflicted with Schizophrenia because their behaviors may seem odd and even bizarre. However, the vast majority of patients who have Schizophrenia are fully able to converse normally about everyday matters even if they seem a bit distracted at times. A physician, family member or friend can often strike a peaceful co-existence between the patient's "inner world" and the "real world" with which these patients are also in touch. After a while, I will ask patients to report on the events in their "outside" world, meaning their real life, and then, I will also ask about the happenings in their "inside" world. Although I am interested in the general content and tone of the patient's inner world, I convey over time to them that, while seeming very real to them, it is a manifestation of their sickness. Because of the chronicity and the isolation resulting from the nature of this condition, it is appropriate and recommended that these patients be in long term supportive care with meetings on the order of once a month even if the symptoms are stable. This need not be done by the psychiatrist who could see the patient less often.

Supportive care is warranted in order for the patient to have regular contact with someone who can maintain a stable contact with the person behind the illness.

My standard advice to patients who are actively having psychotic experiences, such as delusions (false beliefs) and hallucinations (hearing voices), is that they should attempt to ignore them. I tell patients that these manifestations of the illness "feed on" the patient's involvement in them, and if they can be "starved" of this attention, they will tend to fade. This is the kind of advice that is impossible to fully really follow, but it gives the patient something to do which is in the "right direction." I think that a more organized Cognitive Therapy approach in which the hallucinations and delusions are systematically challenged is a valid psychotherapeutic approach when presented as a "coping tool" and not a cure. A healer must be cautious about overselling treatments which require "homework," such as keeping records of their inner life, etc., lest their failure leave the patient with a feeling of even further inadequacy.

Medications are almost always indicated in the treatment of Schizophrenia and, therefore a psychiatrist should be the central figure in the team. Antipsychotic medication for Schizophrenia has been available since the discovery of Thorazine (available as chlorpromazine) over 50 years ago. These medications, also called "Major Tranquillizers" are able to calm the hyperactive, psychotic mental process without rendering the patient unconscious and asleep. Nevertheless, early in the treatment of severe psychosis, it is often therapeutic for the patient to be either asleep or adequately sedated most of the first several days. The comparison of using a splint for a fractured bone is validly invoked. The brain must be "held still" for a while so it can knit together and heal. These and the newer so-called Atypical Antipsychotic medications all have serious side effects which shall be discussed, but their benefits must be stressed first.

There is wide agreement in the psychiatric and patient community that the benefits derived from controlling an actively agitated psychotic state outweigh the risks involved in taking these medications. Although somewhat more controversial, chronic administration of these medications is often necessary in order to prevent a relapse. Anyone who spends enough time around acutely mentally ill patients, including the overwhelming majority of patients themselves, becomes a believer that relief from this dreadful suffering is worth considerable risks. To me the necessity to treat these conditions arises from common sense. Once again, the symptoms of acute mental illness manifest a breakdown of function and are not part of any purposeful behavior, such as trying to get attention, or, as some have suggested with respect to Schizophrenia, a vestige of some prehistoric "soothsayer" role; rather, they are the result of large portions of the brain escaping from their regulatory mechanisms into uncontrolled hyperactivity in much the same way cancer grows unabated without treatment. It just makes sense that being in these hyperactive mental states for long periods of time is highly toxic for the brain in ways which we are only beginning to understand. As stated in the introduction, most of the disordered changes in the physiology of mental illness are the effects of these diseases, not their causes. Generally speaking, the more time one spends in any mentally ill state, the higher the risk for recurrence of that illness in the future. It is as if pathological neuronal pathways for the illness are being progressively established as long as it is active.

As important as antipsychotic medications are, patients, family and friends should be aware of their side effects. These Major Tranquillizers can be divided into the original group which followed Thorazine, including Mellaril, Trilifon, Haldol (all available in generic form) and others now referred to as "Classical Antipsychotics," and a newer group, including Risperdal (available as risperidone), Zyprexa (generic: Olanzepine), Seroquel (generic quetiapine), Geodon (generic: ziprasidone), Abilify (generic: aripiprazole), and Fanapt (generic: iloperidone), called "Atypical Antipsychotics." The difference between these two groups of medications is not primarily in their basic effectiveness in treating the illness, but in their side-effect profile. The two basic problematic side effects caused by the Classical Antipsychotics are symptoms of Parkinson's Disease and a movement disorder called Tardive Dyskinesia. The Parkinson's side effects most noticeably include characteristic stiffness in the walking gait with absence of normal arm swinging, hand tremor, and decreased facial mobility ("mask-like facies"). These symptoms are reversible after the medication is stopped. Tardive Dyskinesia is not as common as the Parkinsonian effects, but its incidence increases with the accumulated time on the medication, and may not fully reveal itself until the medication is lowered or stopped. The problem consists of a periodic writhing or twisting movement most commonly in the mouth or tongue Of most concern is that, once it appears, it can be difficult to treat and can last for many months or even years after the medication has been discontinued.

Because of these side effects in the Classical Antipsychotic medications, it was with great positive anticipation that the new generation of Atypical Antipsychotics was received. The most significant change is decreased incidence of Parkinsonism and lowered risk (not zero) of Tardive Dyskinesia, with variations amongst these medications. Furthermore, in addition to reducing the intensity of hallucinations and delusions, these newer drugs appear to improve depression including the so called negative, symptoms of Schizophrenia. These medications, most particularly Zyprexa, are extremely well tolerated in the short run, meaning days to weeks, for the acute, agitated psychotic episodes.

But, alas, these medications have another set of problems, particularly when used for months or years. Zyprexa and Seroquel have a marked tendency to cause frequently alarming weight gain. This problem can with difficulty be counteracted by a strict regimen of diet and exercise which needs to be persistently encouraged. Risperdal, Geodon and Abilify cause substantially less weight gain. Of most concern with these newer drugs is their tendency, somewhat independent of the weight gain effect, to precipitate diabetes in patients who are predisposed to it. These medications have also been linked to increases in cholesterol and lipids in the blood, which, in turn, are linked to heart disease. All this means that patients on these medications must be closely monitored with blood tests and measurements of girth and weight.

The principal tragedy of Schizophrenia is disability in the area that makes life most meaningful and from which life's greatest comfort lies: the closeness of communal feelings in relationships. I have had many conversations with patients about this topic, most of whom are all too aware of the isolation imposed by their condition. Suicide is not infrequently a risk when this reality first hits home. Nevertheless, it is with great courage that many of these patients and, most especially their friends and family, grow to accept these limitations and go on to share their lives.

Schizophrenia reveals the unique world in which we live by means of its profound disruption within the mind of those who suffer from this condition. As I have spent countless hours in the company of patients with Schizophrenia, I have come to appreciate the miracle of the symbolic world into which, in health, we humans are delivered as I have watched it sucked into a distorted vortex by this illness. We take for granted the grandeur of this social apparatus because it is the very air we breathe with one another and the very water in which we swim together.

Chapter 11

DEMENTIA

The only "Law" in psychiatry states that any possible physical, organic cause of psychiatric symptoms should be considered and treated first, or at least concurrently, pertains to patients with dementia. Nevertheless depression, anxiety and personality changes are, of course, very much part of these disorders. Most of the neurology in our brains is inhibitory to the unique combination of emotions that comprise the "engine" of our personalities. As the neurological restraining and modulating effects are disabled by dementia, a caricature of the patient's personality often emerges in "bas relief." Previously enterprising, type A personalities might become frustrated and angrily resist, for example, the idea that they cannot drive. A shy person might become withdrawn, a demanding person, more demanding, and an anxious, insecure person might become paranoid.

Inevitably, a neurological function that is progressively worn away is that which can react to how other people are reacting. This central feature, the lessening of the ability to empathize with other people's responses, results in the painful reality of progressive emotional separation from friends and family. Sometimes the patient responds to this emotional separation with increased anxiety, or by demanding constant contact with the partner. In order to preserve the functioning and mental health of the patient's spouse, it often is important, with the help of other caretakers if necessary, to advise regular outings away from the patient including socializing with friends.

Alternatively, it may be the case that other patients are spared the suffering of being aware of their increasing disabilities. If so, it is sometimes therapeutic for friends and family to be encouraged to analyze carefully their own assessment of the subjective suffering of the patient. It is natural to react to those who have an illness by transposing oneself into the patient's circumstance and thus to imagine the experience of dementia as being trapped within a horrific prison. But this reaction often does not take into account the merciful diminishment of the universe of the patient's own awareness in both space and time to, perhaps, a circumference of several feet or even inches, and a span of several minutes or even seconds.

The treatment of the psychiatric symptoms that frequently accompany dementia is similar to the treatment of symptoms in Post-Traumatic Stress Disorder. The treatment is purely symptomatic in that the medications are chosen on the basis of the symptoms that predominate at the time. If anxiety or depression predominates, SSRI antidepressants are used. If the depression is more of the shutdown variety with lack of initative and lethargy, one of the more stimulating antidepressants, such as Wellbutrin (generic: bupropion), or, perhaps, a stimulant such as Provigil (generic: modafinil — a medication approved for narcolepsy), or even small amounts of Ritalin (available as methylphenidate) or Dexedrine (available as dextroamphe-tamine) might be used.

Because the neurological circuitry that is being damaged in dementia is mainly inhibitory, the result is commonly a release into hyperactivity and agitation. Whereas in mental illness discreet emotions or functional subsystems are released into feedback reverberation, in dementia the breakdown into hyperactivity often cuts across these diagnostic categories resulting in a more neurologically wide-spread agitation, which is extremely difficult to treat. Further complicating the treatment of agitation in dementia is the constantly changing nature of the problem as a result of the progression of the disease. Virtually every medication in the psychiatric armamentarium with a remotely calming effect may be validly given a trial in intransigent cases of agitation in dementia. The problem is that the effectiveness of these medications is notoriously inconsistent for controlling agitation in this patient population. In short, it is a "hit or miss" proposition and the treating physician may have to keep changing medications in response to constant changes in the patient.

In general, the physician may start with very small doses, work up slowly, and continue making small changes both up and down in response to frequent reports from family, friends or other caretakers. Shorter acting benzodiazepine tranquilizers like Ativan (available as lorazepam); anticonvulsants, such as Depakote and Neurontin (available as gabapentin) can be helpful. Antipsychotic medication is used with special caution in dementia. In addition to over-sedation and the risks detailed in the chapter on Schizophrenia, there are statistical indications of a slight but significant increase in the incidence of stroke and mortality in general incurred by the use of these medications in this population. The risk of falling is ever present. However, the critics of medicating these patients would be surely be tempered by day in and day out exposure to chronic, sometimes combative agitation in a family member. This is a situation in which there must be close collaboration between physician and family in assessing the level of agitation in the patient and open discussion as to the pros and cons of increasing, decreasing or changing the medication.

For families with a relative suffering from dementia, it is common for them to feel that nothing seems to be right, something is always going wrong; their reactions have been too harsh or not responsive enough, the setting too unmonitored or too restrictive. Dealing with Dementia is frequently an extremely messy process in which nothing seems to work out well, leaving everyone exhausted. The candle of the patient's spirit is cast out into a stormy sea that tears apart its ship through which its flicker is diminishingly glimpsed. Then, when it is over, commences the healing process of reclaiming and reinstalling into the family the vital person who existed before the illness with the reconstruction of this spirit to guide the younger generation forward.

Chapter 12

FINAL COMMENT FROM THE AUTHOR

This guidebook revived the venerable idea that mental illnesses centrally occur as dysfunctions of dynamically interacting emotions. Illness occurs when normal emotional functions spin out of control into a self-sustaining state of hyperactivity, which I have called feedback reverberation, a process that then, secondarily, is instantiated at the molecular level of the brain. The brain's own defense against this painful and toxic feedback reverberation state is depression, the essence of which is the disengagement of all motivation to do anything. Like many of the body's defenses against illnesses, such as fever or inflammation, etc., depression often does not "work" in settling down the emotional hyperactivity and creates its own symptoms, adding insult to injury. All treatments for mental illness, including psychotherapy, medications and even electroconvulsive therapy are attempts to slow down and re-regulate hyperactive emotional circuitry so that, in the case of depression, the brain no longer needs to shut down in response to it.

Once diagnosed, the most important advice for family, friends, and, most of all, for the patient him or herself is to grant the illness the status accorded to physical sicknesses. This means that the normal occupational and social demands on the patient should be suspended in return for the patient's actively seeking help from professional care-givers. Family and friends are encouraged to give deference and respect in acknowledgment that the patient is in a state of painful suffering in return for which the patient acknowledges that, beyond emotional support and advocacy, that there is nothing decisive they, themselves, can do.

The most important subtext for the mental health caregiver to constantly purvey is that almost all mental illnesses eventually improve with persistent efforts at treatment. Do not give up, and do not settle for the patient getting only a little bit better. If progress seems to be stalled, seek other opinions and employ simultaneous modalities of treatments. It is almost always more effective for serious, intransigent psychiatric problems to be treated by both medications and psychotherapy.

INDEX

About the Author

John V. Wylie received a bachelor of arts degree from Yale University, an M.D. from Columbia University College of Physician and Surgeons, and then obtained his psychiatric training at Georgetown University Hospital, with which he continued to be associated on the clinical teaching faculty. He practiced general psychiatry in Washington, D.C., where he was on the medical staff at Sibley Memorial Hospital, serving as Chairman of the Department of Psychiatry from 1988 to 1995. Now retired, he lives and writes in Olney, Maryland, with his wife, Ann, and German Shepherd, Tulip.